BINGE BRITAIN

D0265595

BINGE BRITAIN
Alcohol and the National Response

Martin Plant
Moira Plant

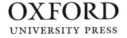

OXFORD
UNIVERSITY PRESS

OXFORD
UNIVERSITY PRESS

Great Clarendon Street, Oxford OX2 6DP

Oxford University Press is a department of the University of Oxford.
It furthers the University's objective of excellence in research, scholarship,
and education by publishing worldwide in

Oxford New York

Auckland Cape Town Dar es Salaam Hong Kong Karachi
Kuala Lumpur Madrid Melbourne Mexico City Nairobi
New Delhi Shanghai Taipei Toronto

With offices in

Argentina Austria Brazil Chile Czech Republic France Greece
Guatemala Hungary Italy Japan Poland Portugal
Singapore South Korea Switzerland Thailand Turkey Ukraine Vietnam

Oxford is a registerd trade mark of Oxford University Press
in the UK and in certain other countries

Published in the United States
by Oxford University Press Inc., New York

British Library Cataloguing in Publication Data

Data available

Library of Congress Cataloging in Publication Data

Data available

Typeset by SPI Publisher Services, Pondicherry, India
Printed in Great Britain
on acid-free paper by
Biddles Ltd., Kings Lynn, UK

ISBN 0-19-9299404   978-0-19-9299409 (Hbk)
ISBN 0-19-9299412 (Pbk.)   978-0-19-9299416 (Pbk.)
1 3 5 7 9 10 8 6 4 2

The Authors

Martin Plant is Professor of Addiction Studies at the University of the West of England, Bristol. He is also Director of the Alcohol & Health Research Trust, a charity. His publications include the books *Drugtakers in an English Town, Drugs in Perspective, Risktakers: Alcohol, Drugs, Sex and Youth, Alcohol: Minimising the Harm* and *the Alcohol Report.* He is Director of the UK part of the European School Survey Project on Alcohol & other Drugs (ESPAD).

Moira Plant is Professor of Alcohol Studies at the University of the West of England, Bristol. She is also Director of the Alcohol & Health Research Trust. Her publications include the books *Women, Drinking and Pregnancy, Risktakers: Alcohol, Drugs, Sex and Youth* and *Women and Alcohol: Contemporary and Historical Perspectives.* She is Director of the UK and Isle of Man components of Gender, Alcohol & Culture: an International Study (GENACIS).

Acknowledgements

Many people have helped in the production of this book. These include our daughter, Emma Plant, who played a major role in writing Chapter 6. Professor Gerry Stimson and Dr Tim Rhodes are thanked for permission to publish material in Chapter 6 that, at the time of writing, was in press for the *International Journal of Drug Policy*. In addition, information and advice have been provided by the late Dr Christopher Clayson, Dr Douglas Cameron, Professor Christine Godfrey, Dr Kathryn Graham, Ms Joanna Green, Dr Tom Greenfield, Mr Larry Harrison, Professor Nick Heather, Dr James Kneale, Professor Roy Light, Mr Ron McKechnie, Dr Patrick Miller, Dr Hildigunnur Olafsdottír, Mr Richard Pates, Mr Robert Phipps, Professor Robin Room, Professor Tim Stockwell, and Mr Andy Tighe. The production of this book has been generously supported by the University of the West of England, Bristol. Ms Alena Macevoy is thanked for producing a number of figures and graphs. Mr Adrian Guy, Ms Liza McCarron, and Mr Ian Parsons are thanked for rescuing us from several technical problems and providing vital help. Mr David Watkins is thanked for photographs. The Office of Public Sector Information and TSU are thanked for permission to reproduce Crown copyright information. The authors' past research has been supported by many agencies. These include the University of the West of England, Bristol, charities, research councils, the beverage alcohol industry, government departments, health care trusts, local authorities, the police, universities, the European Union, and the World Health Organization. The views expressed in this book are those of the authors. They do not necessarily represent any of the agencies that have ever funded their work.

Contents

Introduction

'Binge drinking' has hardly been out of the news for months. Countless newspaper, radio, and television reports have given graphic details of the effects of this phenomenon. What is binge drinking? Is it new? Is it uniquely British and what can we do about it? This book provides a user-friendly guide to some of the historical, contemporary, and practical issues related to the way we drink in Britain.

Beverage alcohol is widely and approvingly consumed in most, though not all, societies. Alcohol is a molecule consisting of one carbon and two hydrogen atoms. Science apart, vast numbers of people simply like the taste and effects of drinks containing alcohol. Alcohol, originally an Arabic word, is another term for ethanol, or ethyl alcohol. This is made by the fermenting of foods such as barley, hops, and grapes. Other types of alcohol include methanol, isopropyl alcohol, and ethylene glycol. The latter are poisonous. Beverage alcohol is a substance that depresses the nervous system. It produces intoxication because of its action on the brain. Alcohol consumption is generally enjoyable. Even so, heavy and inappropriate drinking is associated with a constellation of dose-related adverse effects.

The consequences of consuming alcoholic beverages are by no means all bad. Most people who drink generally do so in moderation and enjoy the taste and effects of alcohol. The effects of drinking are considered in Chapter 3. It should be emphasized at the outset that alcohol is a psychoactive (mind-altering) drug. Its popularity and chemistry combine to make it one of humanity's biggest sources of both pleasure and pain.

What is a binge?

The term 'binge drinking' (sometimes called 'bout drinking') has been used to denote 'excessive,' immoderate, or heavy drinking. In fact this term has been used in two distinct ways. The first has been used by psychiatrists and other health professionals to describe a 'bender,' a prolonged drinking spree during which an individual drinks in a sustained manner and gives up other activities for at least two or three days. Kessel and Walton (1965, p.90) described this phenomenon in these words:

'There are people who for three or six months, and sometimes longer, drink only socially, if at all. They then suddenly drink excessively for days on end, drinking all the time, neglecting all their responsibilities at work or to their families.'

The second and increasingly popular meaning of the term 'binge' relates to a single drinking session intended to or actually leading to intoxication. This session need not be prolonged but is assumed to be at least potentially risky. The latter use of the expression 'binge drinking' has been very common in the recent popular discussion about heavy and problematic alcoholic consumption in the UK, the USA and elsewhere as well as in the current academic literature. Weschler *et al.* (1994) in the USA used the term 'binge' to describe the consumption of five 'standard' drinks in a row by male students and four drinks in a row by female students. Several commentators have noted that there is no particular reason why four or five drinks in the USA need be a special cut-off point for either alcohol consumption or its consequences. (It should be noted here that a standard USA drink contains 12 grams of alcohol, while a UK unit or standard drink officially contains only eight grams. In fact many British servings of wine and spirits are far more generous than this. In addition, some beers and wines are much stronger.) A unit is equal to a small glass of wine, a pub measure of spirits or half a pint of 'normal' strength beer, cider, lager or stout.

Until recently the editors of the prestigious *Journal of Studies on Alcohol* attempted to hold the line in defence of the traditional, clinical, meaning of a binge:

'To most people, binge drinking brings to mind a self-destructive and unre-strained drinking bout lasting for at least a couple of days during which time the heavily intoxicated drinker 'drops out' by not working, ignoring responsibil-ities, squandering money, and engaging in other harmful behaviors such as fighting or risky sex. This view is consistent with that portrayed in dictionary definitions, in literature, in art, and in plays or films such as the classic *Come Back Little Sheeba* and *Lost Weekend* or the recent *Leaving Las Vegas*.

It is also consistent with the usage of physicians and other clinicians. As the editor of the *Journal of Studies on Alcohol* emphasizes, binge describes an extended period of time (typically at least two days) during which time a person repeatedly becomes intoxicated and gives up his or her usual activities and obligations in order to become intoxicated. It is the combination of prolonged use and the giving up of usual activities that forms the core of the clinical definition of binge. Other researchers have explained that it is counter-productive to brand as pathological the consumption of only five drinks over the course of an evening of eating and socializing. It is clearly inappropriate to equate it with a binge. A recent Swedish study, for example, defines a binge as the consumption of half a bottle of spirits or two bottles of wine on the same occasion. Similarly, a study in Italy found that consuming an average of eight drinks a day was considered normal drinking—clearly not bingeing. In the UK, bingeing is commonly defined as consuming eleven or more drinks on an occasion. But in the USA, some researchers have defined bingeing as consuming five or more drinks on an occasion (an 'occasion' can refer to an entire day). And now some have even expanded the definition to include consuming four or more drinks on an occasion by a woman.

Consider a woman who has two glasses of wine with her leisurely dinner and then sips two more drinks over the course of a four or five hour evening. In the view of most people, such a woman would be acting responsibly. Indeed her blood alcohol content would remain low. It's difficult to imagine that she would even be able to feel the effects of the alcohol. However, some researchers would now define her as a binger!

How useful is such an unrealistic definition? It is very useful if the intent is to inflate the extent of a social problem. And it would please members of the Prohibition Party and the Women's Christian Temperance Union. But it is not very useful if the intent is to accurately describe reality to the average person.

It is highly unrealistic and inappropriate to apply a prohibitionist definition to describe drinking in the USA today. Perhaps we should define binge drinking as any intoxicated drinking that leads to certain harmful or destructive behaviours. Perhaps we should at least require that a person have a certain minimum level of alcohol in the bloodstream as a prerequisite to be considered a binger. Perhaps we could even require that a person be intoxicated before being labelled a 'binger.' But one thing is certain: the unrealistic definitions being promoted by some researchers are misleading and deceptive at best. The conclusion is clear: 'Be very sceptical the next time you hear or read a report about "binge" drinking. Were the people in question really bingeing? By any reasonable definition, most almost certainly were not.' (*Journal of Studies on Alcohol* online)

During November 2003 a symposium in Washington DC was convened to discuss the controversial use and definition of the term 'binge'. This meeting was attended by one of the authors (Martin Plant). As the result of this meeting the National Institute on Alcohol Abuse and Alcoholism (NIAAA)(USA) produced the following definition:

'NIAAA defines a 'binge' as a pattern of drinking alcohol that corresponds to consuming five or more drinks for a male or four or more drinks for a female in about 2 hours. A 'drink' refers to half an ounce of alcohol (e.g. one 12 oz. beer, one 5 oz. glass of wine, one 1.5 oz. shot of distilled spirits). For some individuals (e.g. older people; those taking other drugs or certain medications), the number of drinks needed to reach a binge-level blood alcohol content is lower than for the 'typical adult.'

NIAAA also notes that 'A drinking binge is a pattern of drinking that brings blood alcohol concentration (BAC) to 0.08 or above.'

An interim analytical report by the UK Prime Minister's Strategy Unit (2003) defined a 'binge' as drinking over twice the UK recommended daily guidelines for low risk drinking in one day. This is equivalent to six 'units' for females and eight or more 'units' for males. A 'unit' is equivalent to one centilitre or 7.9 grams of alcohol. This approximates to a single bar room measure of spirits, half a pint of normal strength beer, lager, or cider or a small glass of wine. It should be noted that national standard drinks or 'units' vary. Many British bars now serve measures of spirits that are larger than the traditional one. In addition, glasses of wine are served in many sizes, not least when served in people's private homes. A daunting variety of beverage types (over 4000) are now available with widely differing strengths. Beers range from low alcohol drinks with an alcohol by volume (ABV) of less than 0.1% to brands such as Carling Black Label at 4% ABV (2.25 units in a pint) and strong ales with an ABV exceeding 9% (e.g. the aptly named 'Skull Splitter Ale' with 4.75 units per pint). Wines commonly vary in strength from 10–13% ABV and spirits are often in the region of 37–40% ABV A one litre bottle of a popular supermarket's Scotch Whisky, for example, contains 40 units of alcohol (Alker 2004). To confuse the picture even further, the size of a 'standard drink' varies internationally. A US standard drink is 12 grams, equal to 1.5 UK units. A Canadian standard drink is 13.6 grams, while in Australia and New Zealand it is 10 grams. In Japan, remarkably, it is 20–23 grams (Stockwell and Single 1997, Anzai 2005). The Strategy Unit noted (p.11):

> '... binge drinking is a debated term. Since alcohol will affect people in different ways, there is no fixed relationship between the amount drunk and its consequences. So although many people understand 'binge' to mean deliberately drinking to excess, or drinking to get drunk not everyone drinking over 6–8 units in a single day will fit into this category. Similarly, many people who *are* drinking to get drunk will drink far in excess of the 6–8 unit-based definition.'

To add to the confusion, a Home Office report by Mathews and Richardson (2005) employed yet another way of defining binge. These authors defined binge drinkers as people who reported having felt 'very drunk' once or more in the past 12 months. This strange definition ignores the fact that recent scientific studies have defined a binge in terms of specific and objective quantities of alcohol.

The term 'binge' is sometimes used in this book because this expression is now in general use both in the UK and elsewhere. Even so, it would be better in some ways to use the term 'heavy episodic drinking' since this gives a clearer impression of what is meant. Later in this book a review of some of the evidence about drinking patterns and the consequences of drinking is provided. This describes alcohol consumption, whenever possible, in more precise terms.

Chapter 1

Alcohol in Britain

A Long Time Ago

Excuses for Drinking

Some drink to make them wide awake,
  And some to make them sleep;
Some drink because they are merry,
  And some because they weep.

Some drink because they're very hot,
  And some because they're cold;
Some drink to cheer them when they're young,
  And some because they're old.

Some drink to give them appetite,
  And some to aid digestion;
Some, for the doctor says it's right.
  And some without a question.

Some drink when they a bargain make,
  And some because of loss;
Some drink when they their pleasure take,
  And some when they are cross.

Some drink for sake of company,
  While some drink on the sly;
And many drink, but never think
  About the reason why.

(Temperance Poem 1880s)

Alcohol has played a major part in British life for centuries. It has led to the rise and fall of governments, financed wars, provoked civil disorder and even acts of terrorism. Alcohol, the favoured drug of much of humanity, has a very long history. Early human ancestors such as the australopithecines, living in Africa 3–4 million years ago possibly experienced the intoxicating effects of alcohol when they consumed rotten, fermented fruit. They may have enjoyed it and sought it out as some modern apes and other animals such as elk (moose) and elephants do (e.g. BBC News Online 1999, Harding 2005). Most of us do the same. Archaeological evidence shows that people have been making and consuming alcohol for at least 7000 years. Mesopotamian texts from 5000 years ago make frequent reference to a variety of types of beer. It was clearly being produced on a large scale at this time. Drinking to the point of intoxication and beyond is certainly not new. In fact 'drunkenness' has been recognized as a major social problem in many cultures for thousands of years. This fact has been documented and discussed in an extensive and fascinating literature (e.g. Pitman and Raskin-White Heath 1995, 1991). Attempts to control access to alcohol have ancient origins—the regulation of drinking houses dates back to the time of ancient Babylon, nearly 3000 years ago, and age restrictions on the consumption of alcoholic beverages were in existence at the time of Plato, over 2000 years ago.

Andrew Barr has written that just as the Inuit have many words for snow, the English language is rich with expressions for being drunk (Barr 1995). Alcohol consumption is so closely integrated into our society that the invitation 'what would you like to drink?' is normally assumed to mean 'what kind of alcoholic beverage would you like?' As outlined in Chapter 2, the overwhelming majority of British adults drink alcohol at least occasionally. It is a commonplace accompaniment of having a good time. Wine has long been integrated into Judeo-Christian religious ritual in relation to Shabbat, Passover, and Communion. Most young people out on a date consume alcohol and it is widely accepted equation that:

Alcohol + Woman = Sex

This is not a uniquely UK view—it is not even new. Indeed in the times of the Greeks and Romans, Juvenal noted: 'When she is drunk what matters to the Goddess of Love? She cannot tell her groin from her head.' (Purcell 1994 p.200).

The British were established consumers of beer, mead, cider, and imported European wine before the Roman Conquest under the Emperor Claudius in AD 43. A drinking pot discovered at the Neolithic site at Skara Brae in the Orkneys appears to have been used for drinking some form of beer. This site was occupied up to 5000 years ago. Several Bronze Age cups and chalices, clearly for alcohol, have been found in Britain that originate from 2200–1500 BC. It has been claimed that the Pictish heather ale was the first of the British beers. Tribal chiefs were buried with their drinking horns for use in the hereafter. The Roman writer Pliny recorded that the British used beer to make 'light' bread. In Roman Britain a network of roadside tabernae (taverns) were established and numerous. These were primarily for the use of Roman troops, but native Britons liked them and used them too. The Romans maintained order in their British tabernae as a matter of course.

Ethelbert, the Anglo-Saxon King of Kent, attempted to regulate the 'eala-hus' (ale house) in the year AD 616 (Gibbons 2001). During the eighth century St Boniface wrote in a letter to the Archbishop of Canterbury:

'In your dioceses the vice of drunkenness is too frequent. This is an evil particular to pagans and our race. Neither the Franks nor the Gauls nor the Lombards nor the Romans nor the Greeks commit it.'

In AD 747 the Archbishop of York forbade priests in his diocese to venture into taverns. This restriction appears to have had little effect.

It has been said that every British school child knows one date, 1066. They may not be aware of one suggested explanation for the outcome of the Battle of Hastings—William of Malmesbury, writing in the twelfth century, reported that King Harold's English army lost this encounter because they had been drinking heavily before the battle. This led them to fight 'with more rashness and precipitate fury than with military skill'. It should, however, be noted that reports such as this have been strongly disputed: '. . . there is absolutely no truth in the absurd propaganda story that the English spent the night of 13–14 of October carousing and feasting while the Normans spent it in prayer and vigil.' (McLynn 1999 p.216)

John of Salisbury, writing in the twelfth century, described witnessing scenes of 'utter drunken carnage' in the England of his day. The cellars of twelfth century Britain well illustrate the importance of alcohol to the richest:

'In the cellar or storeroom should be . . . pure wine, cider, beer, unfermented wine, mixed wine, claret, nectar, mead . . . pear wine, red wine, wine from Auvergne, clove-spiced wine for gluttons whose thirst is unquenchable . . .' (Amt 1993 p.151)

On an individual level alcohol was sometimes used in the most unethical ways to maintain and ensure a slightly different equation in relation to women:

Alcohol + Woman = Compliance

Christina of Markyate, a young woman who wished to enter into a convent, announced her intention of remaining a virgin. She was eventually convinced to marry; however, she made it clear her wish to remain a virgin and enter a holy life was unchanged. In an attempt to change her mind her parents and husband gave her presents, flattered her, and in exasperation threatened her. All to no avail. Finally at a large gathering in their house they tried something else:

'They hoped that the compliments paid to her and the accumulation of little sips of wine would break her resolution and prepare her body for the deed of corruption . . . Against the favours of human flattery she fixed in her memory the thought of the Mother of God . . . Against the urge to drunkenness she opposed her burning thirst.' (Amt 1993 p.139)

In 1267, King Henry III regulated the price and quality of ale and beer had been officially recorded as the 'second necessity of life in the Assize of Bread and

Ale' (Burnett 1999 p.111). The first record of standardizing of control of alcohol by licensing appears to have been in the late 1400s. Medieval British monks often consumed one or two gallons of ale or wine each day. In fact the church was a major alcohol producer. Some monasteries had massive outputs of alcoholic drinks, especially beer. Priests were instructed to teach women about to marry that they be: '... sober in eating and drinking, for of too much eating and drinking comes much quickening of the fire of lechery.' (Amt 1995 p.89)

It was around this time that concerns began to be raised about the reduction in social controls related to drinking which, up until this point had been the territory of women. Brewing was usually the work of women and when alcohol was consumed in the home or in the home of friends, the women exerted powerful if unspoken control over the behaviour of the men. At this time men, either alone or with male friends, began to drink outside the home in taverns where there were few 'respectable women' to provide the control of drunken behaviour.

In 1552 the crown set out through the Alehouse Act to control alehouses in order to reduce drunken and disorderly behaviour. It is evident that local controls were in force during medieval times. The Alehouse Act forbade the sale of ale by anybody who was not licensed to do so by justices of the peace. The number of alehouses was monitored and sometimes restricted—the number of such establishments in Ripon was halved for example (Webb and Webb 1963). It is important to remember that many of the people who frequented alehouses at this time were men back from serving in whichever war was happening at the time. They were often homeless and much of the trouble relating to drunkenness and disorderliness was due to the fact that these men were used to violence as a way of life.

There have been many ceremonies throughout the ages often started in relation to Church rituals and then developed into secular events. The orgy of the Feast of Fools was, according to Partridge (2002):

> 'a ceremony confined in its celebration to members of the clergy. In the reign of Elizabeth it was finally suppressed, only to be replaced by a secular festival; the election of the 'abbot of Unreason' or 'Lord of Misrule.' (p.82)

However this ritual still included use of the Church where much of the celebrations took place. This is an interesting example of the difficulty of not wishing to take part in such behaviour, again, as noted by Partridge:

> 'Members of the court of the Lord of Misrule have badges, and these the attendants sell to anyone who will: maintaine them in this their Heathenrie, Divelrie, Whoredom, Dronkennesse, Pride and whatnot. Anyone who refuses to play up to them is 'Mocked, and flouted at shamefully.' (p.83).

A common thread throughout many of the most extreme times when drinking was out of control (usually related to celebrations) was the pressure to conform. It is seen in parts of Scotland at New Year when being sober is the abnorm not the norm. It is worth asking how much of the drinking and behaviour of young people on our city streets at the weekend is brought about by the pressure to conform.

There have always been differing views on beverage type. Whisky being described in the *Chronicles of England, Scotland and Wales* in 1578 in the following terms: '... truly it is a souereigne liquor if it be orderlie taken.' (Maclean 2003 p.11).

The Tudors and Stuarts

In the reign of Queen Elizabeth, Sir Walter Raleigh wrote:

> Take special care that thou delight not in wine, for there was not any man who came to honour or preferment that loved it; for it transformeth a man into a beast, decayeth health, poisoneth the breath, destroyeth natural heat, deformeth the face, rotteneth the teeth, and to conclude, maketh a man contemptible, soon old, and despised of all wise and worthy men, hated in thy servants, in thyself and in thy companions; for it is a bewitching and infectious vice.' (Williams and Brake 1980 p.1)

The Elizabethans, however, liked alcohol. Queen Elizabeth I, like many of her contemporaries, often drank two pints of strong beer for breakfast. This does not appear to have been regarded as unusual. There were, however, also concerns about the effects of heavy drinking. Between 1604 and 1627 there were seven acts passed in England to attempt to curb public drunkenness. Elizabeth's successor, King James VI of Scotland and I of England produced a book of sports to draw some of his subjects away from alehouses (Gibbons 2001). Kneale (1999) has noted: 'The same complaints recur from 1600 onwards, focusing on disorder, sexuality, pauperism, and threats to family life.' (p334).

The positive and negative effects of alcohol have been known for a long time, as brilliantly expressed as comic relief by the drunken Porter in Shakespeare's play *Macbeth*, written about 1605.

Macduff: 'What three things does drink especially provoke?'

> Porter: 'Marry, sir, nose-painting, sleep, and urine. Lechery, sir, it provokes, and unprovokes; it provokes the desire, but it takes away the performance: therefore, much drink may be said to be an equivocator with lechery: it makes him, and it mars him; it sets him on, and it takes him off; it persuades him, and disheartens him; makes him stand to, and not stand to; in conclusion, equivocates him in a sleep, and, giving him the lie, leaves him.' (*Macbeth*, Act 2, Scene iii)

James VI's son Charles I was much more abstemious. He drank very little compared to others of the time, one glass of watered down wine with his dinner. The continuing theme of the risk to women if they drink was noted by John Gough. In 1684 he wrote: 'A woman and a glass are ever in danger.' (Keeble 1994 p.76).

It has been suggested that alcohol consumption and its associated problems rise and fall in 'long waves' throughout history (Skog 1986). There have been times when heavy drinking has caused such serious problems that Government action has at last been unavoidable. Eventually, if these problems decline, subsequent generations forget about them and if laws are relaxed, the problems will proliferate once more (Greenfield and Giesbrecht 2005).

The Gin Craze

Government policy has sometimes clearly been an important cause of alcohol problems. During the late seventeenth century taxes on gin were reduced in order to increase demand for this drink. Gin consumption was widely regarded as signifying loyalty to the new Protestant monarch, William of Orange. Gin originated in the Netherlands (Musto 1997). The Distilling Act of 1690 was strongly motivated by the government of William I's wish to fill the vacuum left by the absence of newly-banned French brandy. This act also had the advantage of providing a new market for home-grown corn and enabled a new large scale distilling industry to develop. The unforeseen but rapid consequence of this policy was the infamous 'gin epidemic' of the eighteenth century.

During this period the consumption of cheap gin soared, especially among those on low incomes who purchased their gin from thousands of street sellers or vendors operating unlicensed 'gin shops.' There were 10,000 gin shops in London alone. Between 1707 and 1727 gin consumption doubled. A measure of the level of this consumption is provided by the fact that by the year 1742, the British population of fewer than 7 million people were consuming 19 million gallons of gin annually (Brown 2003).

By the mid 1700s James Boswell, biographer of Samuel Johnson, described a common way of drinking called 'spree drinking' which meant drinking to the point of collapse. Was this the equivalent of our modern binge drinking? At this time, in large cities such as London, many of the men lived in lodgings as they came in from the countryside to find work. This meant that they spent a lot of time, and money, in the public alehouses, now shortened to public houses, where they could also get a cheap, but often good, meal. In urban areas public houses were allowed to remain open all night. The consequences of this were vividly depicted by Hogarth's famously hellish picture of life in *Gin Lane* (1751). This shows a grotesque, snuff-using, drunken mother dropping her baby to its probable death. The woman depicted in Hogarth's etching is reputed to be Judith Dufour. Barr describes the crime:

'In one case that came before the Old Bailey, a young woman named Judith Dufour had a two-year-old child housed in the workhouse, where she had been given a new set of clothes. The mother came to take her out for the afternoon. No sooner was she clear of the workhouse however, than she strangled the child, stripped off the clothes, and threw the naked corpse into the ditch in Bethnal Green. She sold the clothes for 1s 4d, with the money she bought gin'. (Barr 1995 p.190).

Hogarth's etching also shows a young woman pouring alcohol or laudanum down the throat of a baby, a practice which continued into the industrial revolution where mothers had to take their babies to work with them in the mills. To keep the babies quiet they were given alcohol or laudanum. Another practice common at the time was for one woman to look after a number of the children while the other mothers went to the mills or out begging. These women also used laudanum or alcohol to keep the children quiet. Hogarth's etching does not stop there. In fact it shows step-by-step the ways that gin was used at the time. Older children are shown drinking from a jug and while it is clear Judith Dufour's child will soon die, it is also clear that she herself would not have lasted long, as shown by the open coffin.

It was no coincidence that 100 years later gin was still sometimes referred to as 'mother's ruin'. The idea that some beverages were more likely to lead to problems was beginning to take hold as noted by Warner (1994) in a verse comparing the two beverages in the eighteenth century. This verse was used to highlight the differences between Hogarth's two famous engravings *Beer Street* and *Gin Lane*:

'Gin, cursed fiend, with Fury fraught
Makes human race a prey,
It enters by a deadly Draught
And steals our Life away
Beer, happy Produce of our Isle
Can Sinewy Strength impart,
And wearied with Fatigue and Toil
Can cheer each manly Heart.'
(Warner 1994 p. 687)

Hogarth, like many of his contemporaries, was not anti-alcohol. His less famous depiction of life, in *Beer Street* expressed the view that moderate drinking of beer, was perfectly compatible with life in an ordered and civilised society.

The ravages of the gin epidemic have been ably documented in great detail elsewhere (e.g. Dillon 2003, Warner 2003). In brief, the widespread heavy consumption of cheap gin was associated with chronic mass intoxication, drunken violence, disease, alcohol dependence, alcohol-related birth damage to babies, and premature mortality. These ills affected females and males, adults and children. Hannah Wooley, the author of *The Gentlewoman's Companion* noted that a child should not drink much wine or spirits in case:

'...he fall into the bibulous habits of the older generation, he should not be permitted to drink without eating...a dangerous beginning.' (Waller 2000 p.67).

The crimes noted at the time included the following:

'Henry Simpkins of the parish of St. Giles in the fields...indicted for ravishing and carnally knowing Grace Price, a girl of ten years of age, against her will. It appeared the prisoner pickt up the girl and carry'd her to an alehouse where he made her drink, and afterwards carry'd her to an empty house in New Buildings...committed the felony, and gave her the pox.' (Waller 2000. p.72)

Alcohol was also used as a medicine:

'Eighteenth-century obstetricians...could not prohibit alcohol because they needed it as a drug...As a result, obstetrical writers took a ambiguous position ...Edward Foster, a Dublin midwifery professor, stated in a 1781 work that uterine haemorrhage, leading to miscarriage or abortion could result from 'the abuse of stimulants, vinous and other strong liquors' but recommended alcohol as a pain killer during pregnancy and delivery.' (Warner and Rosett' 1975 pp.1397–8)

In eighteenth century Scotland it was not unusual for doctors to see their patients in taverns (Graham 1950). Concerns about the heavy drinking of many women resembled those later expressed during the early twenty first century:

'The woman drinker was a threat. She was a threat to society, to her family and to herself. She was a threat to her husband and children.' (Dillon 2003. p.215).

In 1743 Lord Lonsdale in the House of Lords spoke of the concern about the level of drinking and alcohol related harm in London:

'These liquors not only infatuate the mind but poison the body; they fill not only our streets with madness and our prisons with criminals, but our hospitals with cripples...Those women who riot in this poisonous debauchery are quickly disabled from bearing children, or produce children diseased from birth.' (*Encyclopaedia Britannica* 1911).

There are many examples of the number of women who were now drinking to excess, for example:

'...at a meeting of the Middlesex magistrates in 1830 the chairman said that 72 cases of drunkenness brought up at Bow Street on the previous Monday the majority were women who had been picked up in the streets where they had fallen dead drunk.' (*Encyclopaedia Britannica* 1911).

Interestingly at this time one question that was asked was what were the 'drunkards' addicted to? (The term addiction was in use by this time.) Was it the alcohol or was it the condition of being drunk? This question could well be asked again today.

Initially, the Temperance Movement related to moderation of alcohol consumption with a stress on reduction in the intake of spirits, particularly gin. Later the movement included teaching of temperance in schools, church societies, and youth groups and the welcoming in of women who were beginning to be minimally accepted into the political arena. Importantly it also included the beginnings of a medical interest in the subject of alcohol problems, which until this time had been highlighted only when individuals in the profession took an interest.

Revulsion at the effects of heavy gin-drinking resulted in Gin Acts in 1729 and 1736. These acts imposed huge taxes on the sale of gin. The 1729 Act, for example, raised the excise duty on gin by 1400 per cent. Gin sellers had to pay a massive annual licence fee of £20. This legislation failed to have much impact and in 1736 'prohibition' was introduced in the form of higher taxes and the prospect of severe enforcement. This could have resulted in a huge fall in the level of gin consumption. It did not. In fact these harsh measures had little effect because they were simply not enforced. The continued scale of problems associated with heavy gin-drinking led to the passage of additional Gin Acts in 1743 (the Tippling Act), 1751, 1757, and 1760. As noted by Dillon (2003), it was obvious that 'prohibition' was widely unpopular and was also a failure. During this period the excise authorities only managed to collect the tax on 40 gallons of gin!

These measures were generally resented and there were protest riots prompted by the harshness of the laws. 'Jacobite terrorists' even bombed Westminster Hall (rather ineffectually) in protest against the Gin Act. Cheap gin had become a symbol not only of social unrest, but of revolution. As noted by Graham (1950):

> 'In 1725 Parliament ... enforced an impost, which had been thitherto evaded, of 6d on every bushel of malt. At this tyrannical interference with their favourite drink the people rose in wild indignation. The Jacobites adroitly raised the cry 'No Union, no malt tax, no salt tax!' There were fierce riots in Glasgow.' (Graham 1950 p.526)

Graham suggests it was this increase in tax which began the decline of brewing and increased the consumption of whisky. In 1786 the Scottish Distillery Act was passed which added an extra tax onto whisky exported from Scotland to England (MacLean 2003 p.60). There were clear differences between Scotland and England in the eighteenth century with English army officers saying that 'a Scots funeral is merrier than an English wedding' (Graham 1950 p.54). Historically in Scotland 'a dram' was not the measure it is today but rather a third of a pint (MacLean 2003 p.61). A Scotch pint of ale was equivalent to two English quarts (Graham 1950 p.526). It must always be remembered that alcohol has played a part in the positive health of the country but sometimes this was more myth than reality. For example, in the smallpox epidemic of 1750 in Northern Ireland, children were given Irish whiskey in the belief that this might prevent death from smallpox (Malcolm 1986).

The 1743 legislation was a pragmatic compromise between ineffective 'prohibition' and unacceptable liberalisation. It had become obvious that few people would pay exorbitant taxes or fees. Even so, the Hanoverian government was anxious to placate the grain and distilling industries, to reduce the scale of the problems caused by gin guzzling, and to urgently secure taxes to pay for a European war in support of Maria Theresa. Moderate, but strongly enforced, taxation went some way to attaining three of these four diverse objectives. The tax on gin shops was reduced from the annual £50 that nobody paid to only £1 a year. There was some vigorous parliamentary and non-parliamentary opposition to the repeal of the so-called prohibition. This was motivated by the belief that there should be no compromise on the control of a drug that was the root, so many believed, of the vices and depravity of the gin craze. Even so, it was obvious that prohibition had failed. It had also ensured that the government had little influence on any aspect of the gin trade. A 'middle-way' approach won through, but some believed that this was for the wrong reasons:

'...Madam Geneva (gin) was here to stay. Whatever ills she brought with her. Their priority now was to decriminalise gin and bring the industry back within the law. They even accepted that an industry controlled by respectable and profitable businesses would provide its own form of control... It was a pact with the devil. 1743 would be the peak of the eighteenth century gin craze. From that year onwards, spirit consumption would decline for the next forty years. Not until the mid 1780s would it start to rise again.' (Dillon 2003 p.228).

The medical historian David Musto has commented on the end of the gin craze in terms that could usefully be noted by twenty first century politicians:

'Due to the fine tuning of taxation and success of the anti-spirits campaign after decades of experience with high consumption, the gin epidemic faded.' (Musto 1997 p.16)

Interestingly as time went on Gin Palaces became more elegant. These often very ornate buildings had beautiful stained glass windows and carved wood panelling as well as crystal chandeliers in the finest examples. Some of these finest Gin Palaces, as well as more modest establishments, had unobtrusive, discreet side doors so that women could enter, usually into smaller rooms, which meant they did not have to walk through the male domain of the public bar.

In the eighteenth century the custom of toasting reached its height. Interestingly both men and women were included in this. As noted by Graham (1950) in Scotland:

'When the table was cleared of viands, and the glasses were once more set on the shining mahogany, each person proposed the health of every other person present severally, and thus, if there were ten guests there were ninety healths drunk...There were also rounds of toasts, each gentleman naming an absent lady, each lady an absent gentleman.' (p78).

After this there were the 'sentiments.' This was a clever or poetic phrase or moral. Along with the varying degrees of drunkenness found at different times, there went skilled and clever ways of avoiding drunkenness. A good example of this was the 'deception glass.' This specially made glass was used by the toast masters of the time. They had to take a drink for every toast and so many of them used a glass which to all intents and purposes looked the same as all the others. However, the bottom of the glass was made of very thick glass which meant that the glass looked as full as the others but only contained about a teaspoonful of alcohol. There must have been many times when the toast master was thankful for this trick!

Other ways of avoiding getting too drunk were also noted. Henry Mackenzie an author in the 1780s described a drinking party. He did not want to drink anymore and so he:

'...dropped off under the table among the slain, as a measure of precaution. Lying there, my attention was called to a small pair of hands working at my throat. On asking what it was, a voice replied, 'Sir, I'm the lad that's to lowse the neck-cloths' [i.e. untie the cravats of the guests and prevent apoplexy or choking from vomiting].' (MacLean 2003 p.63)

The Victorian Era

The problems associated with heavy drinking had been evident for centuries. It was, however, only during the nineteenth century that a scientific medical perspective began to emerge in Britain thanks to men like Drs Trotter (1804) and Sullivan (1899). Medical evidence increasingly became one of the factors that have been taken into account in the consideration of Britain's alcohol problem. Robert Chalmers writing in *Traditions of Edinburgh* in 1825 noted:

'Nothing was so common in the morning as to meet men of high rank and official dignity reeling home from a close in the High Street, where they had spent the night in drinking...Intemperance was the rule to such a degree that the exception could hardly be said to exist.' (MacLean 2003 p.47).

Almost twenty years later concern was still being raised. In 1842, the Select Committee on the Health of Towns noted: 'penury, dirt, misery, drunkenness

and crime culminate in Glasgow to a pitch unparalleled in Great Britain'
(MacLaren 1976 p.17).

The Forbes Mackenzie Act of 1853 included sections on closing hours of 11
p.m. to 8 a.m. on weekdays and Saturdays and all day pub closing on Sundays.
However, this was only in Scotland. It was not until the next year that an
equivalent act was passed in England. This proved so unpopular that it was
repealed in 1855. In Scotland the act was simply defied by many and unlicensed premises called 'shebeens' were set up.

Most public and political attention during the early part of the nineteenth
century was focused on gin. The Beer Act of 1830 was passed in the hope that
people could be diverted from gin to beer, ale or cider.

> 'Basically the act freed up the sale of beer. It was designed to curb the powers of
> the big brewers by liberating the market and making life easier for small busi-
> nesses, thereby generating new competition. It reduced the demand for gin,
> boosted the price of cereal crops.' (Brown 2003 pp.114–15).

In fact, this legislation had some obvious ill effects. The resulting falling beer
prices boosted consumption and licensed premises proliferated. Another
46,000 opened within a few years. This roughly doubled the number of
premises that were selling alcoholic drinks. Drunkenness increased. These
unlicensed 'beer houses' were tolerated until 1869 when they were brought
under the control of local magistrates. It was obvious by then that deregulation had not been a success.

> 'Drunk for a penny, dead drunk for two, clean straw for nothing.'
>
> (Shop sign)

The 1869 legislation laid the foundations for the type of licensing controls
that have been in force ever since. The industrialisation of the late eighteenth
and early nineteenth centuries was accompanied by rapid social change
and many social problems. The latter included widespread drunkenness
and alcohol-fuelled violence: this was evident throughout the night in many
towns and cities because alcohol was on sale all night. The historian Storch
(1977) described the function of the nineteenth century pub in these words:

> 'The pub served as an all-purpose service institution in working-class life (pub-
> licans provided much more than mere drink: house of call, toilet facilities, a
> treasury for sick clubs, refuge from the wet and from the wife, dominoes and
> cards, reading matter, food and music).' (cited by Kneale 1999 p.334).

When the nineteenth century opened, the most universal medical view was
that regular use of alcoholic liquors in 'moderation' (without definition)
was conducive and indeed vital for good health and longevity. However, things
were changing in 1871. Leading doctors including Sir James Paget noted:

'The inconsiderate prescription of large quantities of alcoholic liquids by medical men ... alcohol in whatever form should be prescribed with as much care as any powerful drug.' (Wilson 1940 pp.261–3)

One feature that became commonplace in pubs in the nineteenth century was the bar counter. This gained increasing acceptance after 1830, the year of the Beer Act:

'The open or long bar system, the dominant model for organising pub space after 1850, involved one very large room with a long bar serving customers who stood to drink. Marc Giroud sees the bar counter as the most efficient system for rapid drink sales, driven by rapid urban population growth which had outstripped the provision of pubs. Access to the long bar was further increased by the development of promontory and island bars in the 1870s and 1880s, where the bar projects out into the room or forms a free standing circle.' (Kneale 1999 p.335)

(This design, far from becoming outmoded, has been incorporated in many twentieth and twenty first century urban pubs and clubs.)

The Temperance Movement became a powerful force during the nineteenth century. The United Kingdom Temperance Alliance was founded in 1853. The Temperance movement in Scotland started on the west coast, which had close links to the USA where the idea originated. This organization adopted total abstinence (prohibition) as its main objective. In the 1840s, Dick Turner, a well known abstainer inadvertently coined the phrase 'teetotal'. The legend goes that he was talking about total abstinence but he had a speech impediment, a stutter, and so it came out 'tttttt-total', hence teetotal.

Other temperance organisations included the British Women's Temperance Association, the Good Templars, and the Women's Total Abstinence Union. Public support for temperance or prohibition was mobilised by people such as Manchester's Dr Ralph Grindrod, who debated the alcohol issue with a Mr Youill, a brewer, in front of a crowd of 10,000 people. The latter unanimously acclaimed Dr Grindrod as the winner of this encounter. The Temperance Movement, strongly religious in its leadership and sentiments, successfully galvanised middle class opinion. It was closely linked with more general campaigns for social reform when the country was faced by huge problems of inequality and poverty such as the consumer co-operatives which vowed to 'eradicate intemperance and improvidence' (MacLaren 1976 p.131). There were also the organizations such as the Salvation Army, the Boys Brigade, and the Band of Hope, cycling and walking clubs which gave young men options other than the local pub, and family oriented places like the now alcohol-free music halls.

In the 1860s Gladstone started the idea of alcohol licences for general grocer's stores in an attempt to reduce the number of people who went to public houses. By the late 1890s the women in the movement towards tee-totalism were active in trying to stop the grocers' licences, which they believed had greatly increased female drunkenness. The evidence on this was inconclusive. Many campaigners believed that women were more tempted to buy alcohol in a grocer's store where they would not be identified as drinkers. It also allowed them to 'hide' the cost of alcohol in the rest of the shopping. These campaigners asked their members to boycott the stores which sold alcohol, with limited success.

However there were often advantages to the local communities where alcohol was brewed, for example some areas funded the district nursing service which was of great importance, (particularly to the women and children) based on the Swedish 'Gothenburg system'. In 1896 an attempt was made to break the monopoly of the brewers. This was carried out by the People's Refreshment Houses Association. This body:

> acquired existing licensing premises and reformeded them by providing temperance drinks and food as well as beer; they would then be managed as public trusts ... it seemed possible that a successful alternative to the brewer's tied house system had been found. (Burnett 1999 p.132)

Importantly, the Temperance Movement began to give women a voice in the political life of the country, though not so strongly as in the USA. There were links between the women of the two countries. In the 1830s a temperance society for women in Birmingham (England) had a set of commitments that included:

> 'We agree to abstain from all intoxicating liquors, except for medicinal purposes and in religious ordinances. We promise to use affectionate means to induce our husbands, children and relatives to sign the total abstinence pledge. We promise that those of us who are unmarried will not accept the addresses of any man who is not a member of a Total Abstinence Society.' (Winskill Undated p.150)

It should be borne in mind that laudanum was commonly used at this time as a treatment for nervous conditions. It was made of one part wine to ten parts opium. Other restoratives used mainly if not solely by women were tonic wines. Perhaps the most famous manufacturer was the American Lydia Pinkham. Known for her work as a temperance campaigner she was also the maker of Pinkham's Tonic. Pinkham's tonic contained 20.6% alcohol. Interestingly, in 1909, the American Anti-Saloon year book listed the alcohol content of these tonics—for example, Hostetter's Stomach Bitters-contained 44.3% alcohol. This in itself was not surprising; alcohol had been used for centuries as a substance in which other herbs and medicines were 'suspended' to keep them fresh. What is important is the fact that neither Lydia Pinkham nor other tonic makers seemed to see any conflict between their temperance work and their livelihoods. However, many believed strongly that the best drink was plain, cold water.

> 'With banner and with Badge we come
>   An army true and strong
> To fight against the hosts of Rum
>   And this shall be our song
> We love the clear cold water springs
>   Supplied by gentle showers
> We feel the strength cold water gives
>   The victory is ours.'

(The Cold Water Templar, an 1880s Temperance song)

The Temperance Movement has not had much influence in Britain during the past fifty years. Recent debates about alcohol and its associated problems have taken place in a society in which drinking is widely accepted and the main discourse about alcohol problems is a secular one.

> 'The introduction of Sunday morning closing having proved effective, it was extended to weekdays. First, all-night drinking on weekdays was ended by the 1864 and 1865 Public House Closing Acts, which forbade public houses to sell liquor between 1 a.m. and 4 a.m. except to lodgers. Then, in 1872 the Liberal government introduced a Licensing Act which fixed the weekday closing time at midnight in London and 11 p.m. elsewhere.' (Barr 1995, pp. 138–9)

This legislation was aimed solely at restricting the drinking activities of the unruly masses. It did not apply to the haunts of the rich, namely gentlemen's clubs. This conspicuous anomaly was widely resented. Riots ensued in several areas. The governing Liberals lost the General Election of 1874 at least partly because of this resentment. The victorious Conservatives responded to commercial and popular discontent over licensing restrictions with a minor extension of permitted bar opening hours.

> 'We have now 150,000 licensed drink shops in England; 18,000 retail places in London alone. In 1873, the year of unexampled prosperity, the drink bill, which in 1871 was £118,000,000, rose to £140,000,000, so that the high wages were simply squandered in useless drink.' (*Nuts to Crack for Moderate Drinkers* 1870s)

In 1879 the Habitual Drunkards Act provided for retreats licensed by local authorities for people who were defined as 'habitual drunkards'. This Bill went through many amendments before and after this date and it continues renamed to this day. A further act in 1898 prevented the sale of alcohol to the same 'habitual drunkards'. In Scotland the care of people with alcohol-related problems was aided by provision in the Lunacy Acts Amendment Act 1862. This meant that they could be admitted to asylums voluntarily. By the late 1890s these institutions were spread throughout England and Wales charging between 3s 6d and 7s per head per week depending on the geographical area. Many of these retreats or asylums showed a large number of the inmates as suffering from insanity due to excessive drinking.

Public drunkenness was much reduced in London by the Metropolitan Police Act of 1893. This banned bars from opening before 1 p.m. on Sundays. This legislation succeeded in reducing the scale of alcohol-related disorder and other problems. It was subsequently applied to the rest of Britain. The closing of bars on Sundays was introduced in Ireland in 1878 and in Wales in 1881. Many people evaded these bans by drinking in clubs and other places not covered by these restrictions.

During the nineteenth century two detailed and wide-ranging Parliamentary reports examined the problems associated with alcohol. These were the Select Committee of the House of Commons on Public Houses and Morals (the Villiers Report) (House of Commons 1852–1854) and the Royal Commission on Liquor Licensing Laws (the Peel Report) (House of Commons 1896–1898). As noted by Kneale (1999):

> 'These reports consider the internal spaces of the pub, alongside the more standard concerns of licensing, and adulteration. The Villiers Report can be considered to be, in part, a response to questions of morality raised by the liberalisation of the trade and rising levels of alcohol consumption...While the Peel Report is centrally concerned with the licensing system, and with reductions in the number of licenses, it considers pub spaces in more detail than the earlier report.' (p.336)

The Villiers and Peel reports presented evidence that has a familiar ring today. Concerns were expressed about perpendicular drinking establishments' alleged effect of fostering rapid heavy drinking, of the risks to women working as bar maids or drinking in mixed-sex bars, of the excessive number of licensed premises in some urban areas, of the effects of late-night opening on crime and disorder and of the perceived importance of the supervision and control of licensed premises. The minority report of the Peel Committee recommended cutting the number of licensed premises. (Kneale 1999). Kneale has also remarked that:

> 'Three elements stand out in nineteenth century discourses on drinking: the construction of alcoholism; gender and sexuality; and the internal spaces of the pub.' (p.338)

Religion played an important part in the Temperance and Teetotal Movements. Indeed, members of the Christian religion went to great lengths to show that the wine described in the Bible was non-alcoholic. As noted by Burnett (1999):

'Approval of wine posed difficulties for 19th Century teetotallers, who attempted to redraft some 500 Bible references into non-alcoholic forms, usually unfermented grape juice.' (p.142)

'Teetotal reformers developed the 'two wines' theory that Biblical wines were non-intoxicating; in *The Temperance Bible Commentary* (1868). Revd Dawson Burns and Dr Frederick Lees rewrote 493 references in ways favourable to total abstinence.' (p.222)

In the early nineteenth century one of the most powerful additives to alcohol was opium:

'When we consider that four grains of opium are sufficient to double the intoxicating power of a gallon of porter, the article is still cheap enough to be used by the brewer, without subtracting much from his profits.' (Trotter 1813 p.46).

By the end of that century concerns about the adulteration of beer, with various substances was again being raised. The example from Manchester in 1900 was noted by Burnett (1999):

'A mysterious disease variously described as 'alcoholism' and 'peripheral neuritis', broke out in Manchester, and spread to the Midlands; by the end of the year 6,000 cases were reported and 3,000 deaths had occurred, mainly among heavy drinkers. The disease was eventually traced to arsenical poisoning derived from a firm of brewing manufacturers.' (p.124)

As can be seen from the date, this was good ammunition for the Temperance campaigners and social reformers of the time. It is possible that this provided the final push for the Sales to Children Act of 1901. In the late 1890s concern over the risks to children reached a peak and the Intoxicating Liquor (Sales to Children) Act otherwise known as the 'Child Messenger Act' was put on the statute books in 1901. This Act prohibited the sale of alcohol to children under the age of 14 unless it was in sealed vessels. The idea was to prevent children who were sent to the pub for beer for their fathers drinking it on the way home. Amendments to the act meant that by 1908 it became illegal for children under the age of 14 to go into a bar. It also became illegal to give alcohol to a child under the age of 5 unless there was a medical problem and it was therefore prescribed by a doctor.

The World Wars

The outbreak of the First World War prompted the introduction of controls on the operation of public houses. At the beginning of this conflict pubs were open from 5.30 p.m. until late at night:

'The leniency shown to wives of Servicemen sprang naturally from the goodwill towards men serving with the colours...in view of the danger that a conviction for drunkenness might imperil a woman's separation allowance, constables, instead of arresting a drunken woman, would often advise her to go home quietly.' (Carter 1919 p.239)

It was, however, noted that heavy nocturnal drinking led to widespread absenteeism and industrial inefficiency. New measures were motivated by concerns that heavy drinking and drunkenness were undermining the national capacity to meet the demands of the war effort. The Defence of the Realm Act of 1914 drastically reduced permitted bar opening hours to five and a half hours per day. Alcohol taxes were also raised and the buying of rounds and the provision of credit ('running a tab') in bars was banned. This also led to the production of 'Munition Ale' that was much weaker than the pre-war drink. This helped conserve the use of grain which was needed for food.

Wartime politicians, unlike some of their successors, realised the importance of availability and price as effective alcohol control measures. David Lloyd George, an enthusiastic temperance campaigner, declared in February 1915 that: 'drink is doing more damage in this war than all the German submarines put together.' A few months later he famously declared: 'We are fighting Germany, Austria and drink and as far as I can see the greatest of these deadly foes is drink.'

Wartime powers enabled the government to apply special controls on the operation of bars in localities that were particularly important for the war effort. A number of measures were affected in the Carlisle area that provide early twentieth century examples of what would now be regarded as harm minimization. These included selling lower-strength beers, non-alcoholic beverages and food, in more attractive premises with décor and facilities designed to appeal to women. These measures, together with the removal of large numbers of young men by wartime duty or premature death, drastically reduced national per capita alcohol consumption, drunkenness, and alcohol-related liver cirrhosis (Shadwell 1923, Smart 1974).

The controls of 1914 were largely left untouched after the First World War. A Licensing Act was passed into law in 1921. This did not restore pre-war bar opening hours. Instead, it maintained early morning and afternoon bar closing. It did attempt to reintroduce a degree of relaxation, but was unsuccessful:

Its attempted extension of the opening hours was soon overturned by licensing justices, who were under the impression that early closing time would exert the same beneficial effect on public order in peacetime conditions as it had during the war. (Brown 2003 p.141)

Following the creation of the Irish Free State in 1922, Sunday closing was retained in Northern Ireland. A Royal Commission considered licensing during 1929 and 1930 and did not recommend any change in the existing bar opening hours. Brown (2003) cites evidence given to this commission by Sir Edgar Sanders, who was to become Director of the Brewers' Society:

'The present opening hours have met with extraordinary acceptance by the British public...The earlier closing hour has been a reform of the first magnitude for the whole country. The last hour in the evening is always the worst, whatever the period of opening is, and to get the streets cleared at least an hour earlier than used to be the case has been an enormous benefit.' (p.141)

As noted by Clark and Carnegie (2003):

'The Temperance movement had its first roots in the West of Scotland in the nineteenth century as an attempt to combat the serious social problems of heavy drinking...Tearooms flourished at this time of temperance sentiment and were an important recourse for treats as women could enter them quite freely.' (p.135)

However, women often drank in secretive ways to avoid the stigma of being labelled 'a drinker'. This widened the divide between men's public and so-called social drinking, and women's secret and hidden drinking. In the 1930s one Glasgow woman recalled her mother's drinking:

'My mother always took a drink ...I don't mean she sat in the pub all night ...She always liked her tipple and when she got a handbag, she used to like a handbag that could either carry her hymn book and her bible or half a bottle.' (Clark and Carnegie 2003 p.134)

However much difficulty her mother had getting home on a Saturday night— 'we often wondered how she got home'—, her mother 'never missed church on Sunday' (Clark and Carnegie 2003 p.134).

The Great Depression ensured that falling incomes reduced national per capita alcohol consumption to less than half of what it had been at the beginning of the century. Popular fashions, as always, were changing. The milk bar enjoyed a period of mass popularity during the 1930s. This phenomenon provided a temporary alternative leisure focus for some young people who would otherwise have spent more time in pubs. The coffee bar phenomenon of the 1960s had much the same effect.

Around this time, as the women's liberation movement took hold, the idea arose that women's liberation was one of the reasons for increased female drinking. This was not new. At the beginning of the twentieth century, it was said that the increase in women's drinking was due to the emancipation of women. It is interesting how any widening or empowering in the role of women is linked to negative aspects such as increased alcohol consumption. Perhaps it relates back to the views of women's roles and responsibilities by men such as Lord Rosebery, who, in 1902 noted:

> 'Mother's should take greater responsibility for the welfare of their children, wives for that of their husbands. Some women were 'tainted with incurable laziness and distaste for the obligations of domestic life' they produce unpalatable, half cooked meals that drove their husbands out to seek the warmth and cheer of the public house.' (Burnett 1999 p.131)

In 1908 the Scottish Prohibition Party invited the famous American Temperance campaigner, Carrie A. Nation to visit Britain. Nation was famous for her speeches and prayers said in the houses of ill repute in Kansas. She famously posed with a Bible in one hand, an axe in the other. If the prayers did not work, the axe was used for smashing the barrels of beer. She was not impressed by the situation in Glasgow and stated that: 'Scotland was far nearer hell than Kansas'. (King 1993 p.121)

As noted by Brown (2003), it is clear that whereas alcohol and public bars were viewed as threats during the First World War, they were redefined as assets during the Second World War. Largely because of the retention of controls introduced in 1914, alcohol consumption in 1939 was much lower than it had been in earlier times when there was a high degree of social and political alarm about drinking. There were some protests at the start of the war founded upon fears that alcohol consumption would damage the country and the war effort. Nevertheless, this was not the prevailing opinion. The pub was widely regarded as being the focal point of the local community and a haven. It was good for morale and the war effort. Brewers even stressed the nutritional value of their product at a time of food rationing. The pub was seen, not as a hotbed of drunkenness and vice, but as a place to sip a beer and meet other men and women (civilians and those in the armed forces) in a cosy and relaxed setting. Keeping the pubs open was widely viewed as an important symbol of the fact that the Nazis could not destroy the British way of life even in times of austerity. In fact, thousands of pubs were bombed, but the British bravely kept on drinking and ensured that the troops received their vital ration of beer. Even so, there was concern about the behaviour of young women at the time. Admiral Sir Edward Evans of London Civil Defence was so concerned he wrote to the Home Office in September 1943:

> 'Drunken women out on the street, propositioning everyone in sight, misbehaving themselves all over the shop, throwing themselves at blokes. Leicester Square at night is the resort of the worst type of women and girls consorting with men of the British and American Forces. Of course, the American soldiers are encouraged by these sluts, many of whom should be serving in the forces. At night the square is apparently given over to vicious debauchery.' (Burnett 1999, p.131)

Reductions in consumption around this time seemed to have been linked to the availability of other options—for example, in the 1930s and 1940s, among the working class, there was a movement out of old dilapidated town centre housing to modern suburban housing with more space, gardens etc. as well as cinemas, cafes, dance halls, and annual holidays.

Post War drinking

After the Second World War alcohol rationing was abandoned and UK alcohol consumption began to rise. This increase continued until the end of the 1970s, almost doubling in this time. Adding to the availability of alcohol, in the early 1960s supermarkets were able to obtain licences for selling alcohol. The supermarket Sainsbury's was granted a licence in 1962 and others followed including, interestingly, even the co-operative societies which were founded on reputations of temperance.

As the general level of alcohol consumption increased so too did a constellation of adverse effects such as accidents, injuries, alcohol dependence, illnesses, premature mortality, and public nuisance. In response to a rising number of people who were developing alcohol dependence or 'alcoholism', a national network of specialist agencies was established to provide treatment, counselling, and support for such individuals. The Fellowship of Alcoholics Anonymous (AA), an international self-help organisation, was introduced to the UK during the Second World War by US service personnel. AA spread around the country, giving support to thousands of people. In addition a number of specialist 'alcoholism' treatment units or clinics were established from the early 1960s onwards, together with a nationwide network of councils on alcoholism/alcohol. These agencies have continued, though often very poorly funded, to provide help to people with serious, chronic alcohol problems The UK now has a range of counselling and therapeutic alcohol services offering a variety of approaches. These include both abstinent and non-abstinent treatment goals (Heather 1997, UKATT Research Team 2005a,b).

Sunday closing restrictions in Wales had ceased to be very effective after the Second World War. Many people belonged to licensed clubs and could drink therein on Sundays. The 'local option' was introduced in 1961. This allowed people in different areas to vote every seven years on whether or not to open their local pubs on Sunday. The people of South Wales voted for Sunday opening immediately and most of the rest of Wales subsequently followed them. The last local poll on Sunday opening took place in 1996. The last area of Wales to permit Sunday bar opening was the Dwyfor District of Gwynedd. Only 9 per cent of local residents had taken part in this poll. These local options were discarded under the provisions of the Licensing Act (2003) (BBC News Online 2003).

The concerns about rising levels of heavy drinking prompted the setting up of committees to review licensing arrangements in England and Wales (the Erroll Committee) and in Scotland (the Clayson Committee). These two bodies took evidence from a wide range of interested people, including medical practitioners and representatives of various components of the beverage alcohol industry. The latter were by no means all in favour of liberalising existing licensing arrangements. The two committees produced similar recommendations, including extending the hours during which bars were permitted to open and the admission of children into bars under some circumstances (Erroll of Hale 1972, Clayson 1973), but these two reports were greeted with very different responses. The Erroll Report was mainly received with a combination of indifference and hostility. Most publicans in England and Wales were happy with existing arrangements and the report failed to justify making changes because of potential health or social benefits. In addition there was little support for the suggestion that the minimum legal age of alcohol purchase should be reduced in England and Wales. None of the Erroll Committee's recommendations were introduced until 1988. The Clayson Report had a much more rapid and sympathetic response. At the time, Scottish bars were subject to some restrictions such as 10 p.m. closing on weekdays and Saturday, and Sunday closing that were widely unpopular. It was believed that this led to excessive pressure to drink quickly just before the early closing time. Moreover, many Scottish bar patrons prepared for closing time by purchasing carrier bag loads of alcohol, 'the carry oot,' to drink after the bar had closed. These supplies were piled high behind many Scottish bars. Dr Clayson and his colleagues argued forcefully that some relaxation in bar opening arrangements would reduce this excessive pressure to drink. This would, they suggested, lead to reduced rates of drunkenness and other alcohol-related ills. Unlike its English and Welsh counterpart, the Clayson report was largely well received. Some of its key recommendations were introduced by the Licensing Scotland Act (1976). This allowed bars to open until 11 p.m. and also permitted them to open on Sundays. In addition licensing authorities could grant extensions to enable some bars to open during afternoons or later at night. Children were also allowed to enter licensed premises so long as they consumed food and soft drinks in rooms in which alcohol was not served. The 'carry oot' vanished from most bars overnight, or at least became far less conspicuous.

One of the authors (Martin Plant) had the privilege of interviewing Dr Christopher Clayson in April 2003, shortly before the latter reached the age of 100. He attributed the acceptance of some of his committee's recommendations to the fact that they were explicitly designed to reduce the rapid heavy drinking that was evident under Scotland's previously very restricted bar opening hours. He also emphasised that: 'The misuse of alcohol as indicated by the various offences that were being committed was far worse in Scotland than in England'. The recommendations made by his committee were accordingly portrayed as public health and safety measures. He acknowledged that although he believed the reforms had been popular and mainly good, Scotland's alcohol problems had subsequently increased, as they had south of the border. These trends are described in the next chapter.

Alcohol consumption in the UK has continued to rise slowly after falling slightly, then levelling out during the 1980s. This was the decade of a media panic about 'lager louts'. These were portrayed as intoxicated young men whose aggressive behaviour, both at home and abroad, became a symbol of unsavoury behaviour and national shame. Media coverage of the drunken excesses of British youth has continued unabated. Such concerns have been given momentum by cut price air fares for stag and hen party weekends in Europe or encouraging young tourists to 'drink the night away' in places such as Tallinn, Estonia.

The immediate effects of Scotland's extended bar opening hours appeared to be neutral in relation to both public health and crime (Duffy and Plant 1986). In view of this and strong lobbying by FLAG, a campaign for flexible opening hours, the Home Office supported the liberalisation of bar opening arrangements for England and Wales, even though this was opposed by the Royal Medical Colleges and by Alcohol Concern. The latter maintained that this change would increase the health and other ill effects associated with heavy drinking. The Licensing Act of 1988 was passed in spite of such concerns and permitted bars to remain open during the afternoon. It is clear that the majority of people generally drink enjoyably, in moderation and without harm. Nevertheless, the British are both ambivalent and voyeuristic about heavy drinking and its associated ill-effects. Former Conservative party leader William Hague attracted derision by his disputed claim that when younger, he routinely consumed 14 pints a night. This claim was apparently intended to project a macho image as 'one of the lads'. The media periodically go into a feeding frenzy when reporting the alleged alcohol-related excesses and problems of sporting or entertainment stars such as the late George Best, Paul Gascoigne, the late Oliver Reed, and Robbie Williams. The announcement by the singer Charlotte Church that she sometimes drank 10 double vodkas when she 'went out on the lash' or became 'bladdered' was given widespread newspaper publicity. This combined some statements of concern about such heavy intake. Even so, some reports tended to give the impression that their authors rather admired this behaviour.

The British Prime Minister Tony Blair has described heavy drinking, specifically heavy episodic or 'binge' drinking and its associated public order problems as the 'new British disease' (Hetherington and Bowers 2005). In fact the

British Isles' alcohol problems have been noted for over 1000 years. Moreover, the British are not unique in having a predilection for getting drunk. This carousing instinct is shared by the people of several other nations, especially in the north west and centre of Europe. Britain's drinking culture has also been exported to countries such as Australia, Canada, New Zealand, and the USA, even though these countries currently handle it better than the British. In addition, heavy and unhealthy drinking among Russian men has recently contributed to a substantial reduction of their life expectancy (Obote 2005).

A major issue around alcohol is the ambivalence we have about it. This was well described by Judge Noah S. 'Soggy' Sweat Jnr in the US Congress in 1952:

'You asked me how I feel about whiskey. All right, here is how I feel about whiskey. If, when you say whisky, you mean the devil's brew, the poison scourge, the bloody monster that defiles innocence, dethrones reason, destroys the home, creates misery and poverty, yea, literally takes the bread from the mouths of little children; if you mean the evil drink that topples the Christian man and woman from the pinnacles of righteous, gracious living into the bottomless pit of degradation and despair, shame and helplessness and hopelessness, then I am against it with all my power. But, if when you say whiskey, you mean the oil of conversation, the philosophic wine, the stuff that is consumed when good fellows get together, that puts a song in the hearts and laughter on their lips and the warm glow of contentment in their eyes: if you mean Christmas cheer; if you mean the stimulating drink that puts the spring in the old gentlemen's step on a frosty morning; if you mean the drink that enables a man to magnify his joy, and his happiness and to forget, if only for a little while, life's great tragedies and heartbreaks and sorrows, if you mean that drink, the sale of which pours into our treasuries untold millions of dollars, which are used to provide tender care for our crippled children, our blind, our deaf, our dumb, our pitiful aged and infirm, to build highways, hospitals and schools, then certainly I am in favour of it. This is my stand. I will not retreat from it: I will not compromise.'

The perception of alcohol as a medicine has been noted earlier in this chapter. It is still present particularly in relation to certain beverage types. Although wine, particularly red wine has recently been noted as healthy to drink in moderation, this debate is ongoing. One of the most common alcoholic beverages to be noted as medicinal is whisky. Macdonald (1994), describing the Highlands of Scotland states:

'The woman made me a drink of whisky mixed with condensed milk and cream. As she gave it to me she remarked: 'It's not really a drink—more of a tonic really…' Whisky is considered by many people to be a protection against the cold and a good treatment for colds and sore throats.' (p.142)

Rising alcohol consumption and its associated ills led to the production of alcohol strategies for Wales, Northern Ireland, Scotland and, after a long delay, England. These are considered in Chapter 4.

The concept of social need has long been an important part of liquor licensing in Britain:

'Regulation of the sale of alcohol, by local bodies such as the manorial courts, predates Parliament itself. Historically, licensing provisions have sought to regulate quality and price, the manner of sale/consumption and the availability of alcohol. The last of these, availability, is regulated in three ways: statutory control of licensed hours and persons permitted to purchase alcohol, together with justices' discretion as to the number of outlets, through the mechanism of need/demand.' (Light 2005a)

Light cites the Report of the Departmental Committee on Liquor Licensing:

'The policy of restricting the number of retail outlets for intoxicating liquor to the minimum regarded as necessary for the legitimate needs of the population is older than the licensing law itself, although its application by the licensing authorities and its overt support by central government has varied considerably from time to time.' (Erroll of Hale 1972 p.295)

Things have changed recently in a surprising way, as described by Light (2005a):

'Part way through our research we attended a conference at which the head of liquor licensing at the Home Office gave a paper on the matters being considered by the Home Office review. He did not mention need. Asked why need was not to be considered by the review we were told that the matter had already been debated and the view reached that need should be abandoned. The forum was the Home Office Working Group on Licence Transfers.'

Light has also noted:

'At its last meeting, the Minutes from the Working Group's Meeting (7 March 1996), at item 15. read 'Members had submitted written comments on paper WGLT95(10) and these showed agreement that any system of codified grounds for refusal should *not* include a test of "need" ' (underlined in original) (Home Office, March 1996). The end of need?' (Light 2005a)

This change opened the way for the accelerated development of concentrations of licensed premises in town and city centres (Light 1999). This phenomenon is discussed further in the next chapter.

It is clear that alcohol has played a very prominent part in British life for a long time. It is popular and political. The following chapters attempt to provide an overview of drinking patterns, the consequences of drinking, the recent policy debate, and some of the thorny issues related to keeping the adverse effects of alcohol in check.

Chapter 2

Drinking habits: recent patterns and trends

It is clear that the UK has a long tradition of both moderate and not so moderate drinking. Many detailed studies have examined the patterns of alcohol consumption in the UK during the past thirty years. These show that the vast majority of adolescents and adults consume alcoholic beverages at least occasionally, and that most of these people generally drink moderate amounts that do not have harmful effects. Moreover, it is clear from a large international evidence base that most people who drink alcoholic beverages do so because they enjoy the taste and effects of such drinks and because consuming them is a sociable thing to do. The production, distribution, and sale of alcoholic beverages are very important economically and have been for a long time. Chancellor Gordon Brown's 2005 budget estimated that the Exchequer would obtain £7.9 billion from duties on alcohol in the 2004–2005 financial year. This revenue was projected to increase by roughly 4 per cent in the following year.

Is this just a moral panic?

Is recent alarm about 'binge drinking' and the problems associated with heavy drinking just a 'moral panic'? This is a term originally coined by the sociologist Stanley Cohen (1972) to describe a wave of national moral concern about some form of activity regarded as 'deviant' or socially menacing. Cohen first applied this term in relation to mass media coverage of gang warfare between the youth movements of mods and rockers. The term 'moral panic' has been used to imply that lurid and sensational reporting by the mass media, especially the tabloid press, serves to exaggerate and to demonize.

There are certainly times when popular concerns about some issues, often whipped up by the tabloid press, are exaggerated and appear to lead to moral (or immoral) outrage. Sensationalised reports in the UK have related to 'Teddy boys', rock music, drug users, lager louts, paedophiles, and 'hoodies.' (young people who wear hooded jackets). These appear to have inflamed public outrage, or to have been used as excuses for vigilante-type behaviour (in one case a paediatrician's office was attacked because of a misunderstanding of the word paedophile), or hate crimes against members of ethnic or religious minorities. In fact the popular media offer a chronic diet of moral outrage, often oddly combined with blatant titillation. Tabloids do this constantly. A lot of media stories regularly focus upon sexual activity, drinking, illicit drug use or other forms of behaviour. The latter are routinely reported in an ambivalent way. Lurid headlines sell papers. In the case of drinking, there is ample justification for media interest and public concern. Most people in the UK drink alcoholic beverages at least on occasion and the negative effects of heavy or inappropriate drinking are obviously a big problem. The latter has been with us for a very long time. Sometimes media coverage of alcohol issues has simply been cyclical. It is time to do yet another alcohol story, then one on drugs, followed by one about sex... Such stories often come and go with the seasons. Sometimes media interest really does reflect something *real* happening in the world. This and the following chapter attempt to set out some of the factual evidence about recent British drinking patterns and the consequences of the way people in the UK really drink.

It might be helpful to review some of the evidence that is now available on British drinking patterns and how these relate to those in other countries. Firstly, it needs to be noted that per capita alcohol consumption in the UK has been higher in the past (notably during the Middle Ages and the Gin Epidemic) than it is now. Fig. 2.1 shows how consumption has varied in the UK during the past century. As indicated, alcohol consumption fell during the First World War and remained low during the interwar period and the Second World War. It has risen markedly since 1945, reaching a peak around 1980, then falling and then continuing to rise. Per capita alcohol consumption is a useful indication of trends in drinking, but does not in itself tell us much about which people drink what amounts. This type of information has become increasingly available from surveys. The latter are usually based upon people's self-reports of what they have consumed. Reports of this type give a useful, but not necessarily very accurate, indication of alcohol consumption among particular defined groups. Evidence suggests that surveys generally underreport alcohol consumption. This is attributable to some people refusing to take part or being hard to track down, poor recall, embarrassment/guilt, and deliberate evasion. Conversely some studies of alcohol consumption by teenagers and younger people may also be biased by exaggeration. The authors have noted that some young boys claim to have drunk amounts of alcohol that would have killed a mammoth. It is also a problem that drink sizes vary. This is elaborated below. It should, however, be acknowledged that many British surveys have probably provided underestimates of

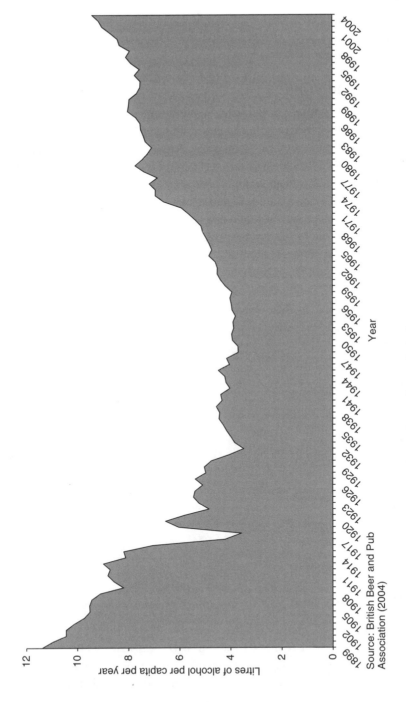

Fig. 2.1 Per capita alcohol consumption in the UK (litres of pure alcohol)

Source: British Beer and Pub Association (2004)

the actual quantities that many people really drink. Accordingly, evidence should be considered overall because this does give a reasonable, if rather vague, picture of what people drink.

Starting to drink

Most young children do not drink and are rather hostile to the very idea. A classic study carried out in Glasgow found children of primary school age to have a negative view of alcohol use, especially that by women (Jahoda and Cramond 1972). Remarkably, a much more recent study of children in Edinburgh and Birmingham found much the same (Fossey 1994). Particular disapproval of women's drinking appears to be deeply rooted in the culture of most, if not all countries where people do drink. The hand that rocks the cradle should not be a shaky one. In spite of this traditional sexist view, it was surprising that children should have still disapproved of women's drinking even though this type of behaviour was by then so commonplace.

Teenagers

The disapproval that many young children have of drinking evaporates with the onset of puberty. Studies have shown for some time that adolescents and teenagers mainly redefine alcohol consumption in a positive way. They regard drinking as being a symbol of maturity and an important requirement of being 'cool,' mature, sexy, and sociable (Davies and Stacey 1972, M.A. Plant et al. 1985, M.A. Plant and M.L. Plant 1992). Most British teenagers are drinking fairly regularly by the ages of 15 and 16 years. Three quarters report that they had been drunk by this age. This is not necessarily illegal. The UK's minimum legal age for alcohol consumption (but not in bars) is only five. Drinking by younger adolescents is often home-based, but becomes increasingly non-home-based as they grow older. Drinking then increasingly occurs away from parental supervision, usually with friends rather than relatives, and often out of doors or illegally in licensed premises. Getting drunk is a normal part of learning about alcohol. Young people report that they begin to drink out of curiosity and to be sociable. There is strong pressure to drink among teenagers.

One study has examined the drinking habits of teenagers across the UK in comparison with those in other countries. The European School Survey Project on Alcohol & other Drugs (ESPAD) was first carried out in 1995 with 29 countries taking part. It has since been repeated in 1999 and 2003 and has grown to include 35 countries or territories (Hibell et al. 1997, 2001, 2004). ESPAD describes the self-reported drinking, smoking, and illicit drug use of representative samples of 15 and 16-year-old school students across Europe. The UK part of this study has shown that UK teenagers are amongst those most likely to report sometimes drinking heavily, being intoxicated, and experiencing adverse effects from their drinking. These adverse effects included individual, delinquency, relationship, and sexual problems.

The latest findings of the ESPAD were published in December 2004. This investigation examined drinking, smoking, and illicit drug use among teenagers in 35 European countries. These included: Austria, Belgium, Bulgaria, Croatia, Cyprus, Czech Republic, Denmark, Estonia, Faroe Islands, Finland, France, Germany, Greece, Greenland, Hungary, Iceland, Ireland, Isle of Man, Italy, Latvia, Lithuania, Malta, Netherlands, Norway, Poland, Portugal, Romania, Russia (Moscow only), Slovak Republic, Slovenia, Sweden, Switzerland, Turkey, Ukraine and the United Kingdom. The overall findings of the 1995 and 1999 ESPAD surveys were generally confirmed by ESPAD 2003. Even so, there were some changes and the inclusion of five new countries also produced a more complex 'map' of teenager behaviours in Europe. In particular, the Isle of Man, the Czech Republic and Switzerland emerged as 'high risk' countries for illicit drug use, with original ESPAD participants, notably the UK and Ireland. 'Binge drinking' was examined on the basis of having consumed five or more drinks in a session on at least three occasions in the previous month. The highest proportions of teenagers who had drunk such amounts were from Ireland (32%), the Netherlands (28%), the UK and the Isle of Man (both 27%). Countries in which such rates were especially low included Turkey (5%), France (9%), Cyprus (10%) and Greece, Iceland, Poland and Romania (all 11%). The levels of 'binge drinking' amongst teenage boys and girls in different countries is shown in Figs. 2.2 and 2.3.

These figures show that in most European countries much higher proportions of boys than girls reported 'binge drinking' in the past 30 days. Even so, as also shown in the figures, comparative information from the Monitoring the Future study by Johnston et al. (2004) in the USA showed that American teenage girls and boys reported equal levels.

The 2003 study confirmed 1995 and 1999 ESPAD findings that teenagers in the UK had high rates of periodic heavy (binge) drinking and illicit drug use. One of the most striking conclusions was the fact that girls in the UK, Ireland, and the Isle of Man were more likely than boys to have consumed five or more drinks at a time, three times or more in the past month. Altogether, 29% of UK girls and 26% of boys had imbibed such amounts (Hibell et al. 2004, M. A. Plant and M. L. Plant 2004, M. A. Plant et al. 2005). ESPAD revealed that only in these countries had girls overtaken the boys in relation to this relatively heavy drinking. In the other 32 survey countries boys remained more likely

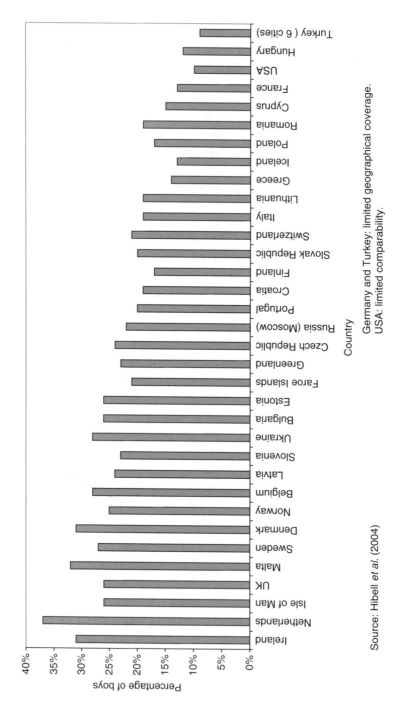

Source: Hibell *et al.* (2004)

Germany and Turkey: limited geographical coverage.
USA: limited comparability.

Fig. 2.2 Proportion of boys (aged 15–16) who reported 'binge drinking' 3 times or more during the last month

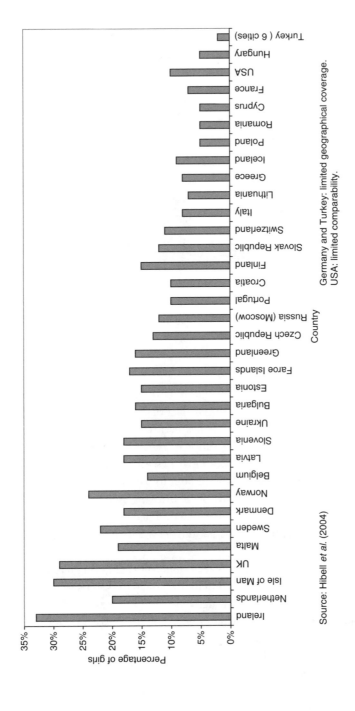

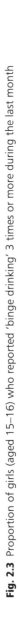

Fig. 2.3 Proportion of girls (aged 15–16) who reported 'binge drinking' 3 times or more during the last month

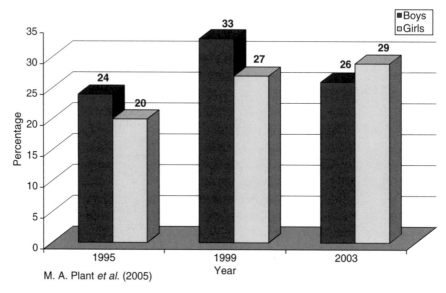

Fig. 2.4 Binge drinking amongst UK 15 and 16-year-olds (1995-2003). Percentage of girls and boys who had consumed five or more drinks at a time, three times or more in the past month.

than girls to have drunk heavily and to have experienced intoxication. This is the traditionally accepted norm. The fact that heavy drinking by UK girls had overtaken boys in some respects has been confirmed by a survey of 11–15-year-olds in England by the National Centre for Social Research and the National Foundation for Educational Research (2005). This indicated that teenage girls were more likely than boys to have been drunk (50% compared with 46%). ESPAD showed that binge drinking among UK teenage boys had risen between 1995 and 1999, then had declined slightly by 2003. In contrast it had risen significantly over the period 1995–2003 in teenage girls. This rise is shown in Fig. 2.4.

A substantial minority of UK teenagers reported having illegally purchased drinks for their own consumption in the past 30 days. Boys were most likely to have bought beer (28%) and wine (20%), while girls were most likely to have bought spirits (25%) and wine (15%). This is consistent with the fact that some UK teenagers reported having consumed their most recent drinks in bars (15% of boys and 18% of girls) or discos (5% of boys and 6% of girls).

Many teenagers in the UK reported that they expected that drinking would produce positive consequences for them. These are elaborated in Table 2.1. Many teenagers also reported expecting that drinking would cause them negative consequences. This is shown in Table 2.2.

Table 2.1 Expected positive consequences of personal alcohol use (percentage of those replying 'likely' or 'very likely')

Positive consequences	Boys (%)	Girls (%)
Have a lot of fun	78	84
Feel happy	74	82
Feel more friendly and outgoing	72	79
Feel relaxed	70	67
Forget my problems	52	55

Table 2.2 Expected negative consequences of personal alcohol use (percentage of those replying 'likely' or 'very likely')

Negative consequences	Boys (%)	Girls (%)
Do something I would regret	39	41
Get hangover	32	34
Harm my health	28	35
Feel sick	26	32
Not able to stop drinking	15	16
Get into trouble with police	19	14

As these two tables show, the great majority of teenagers expected that their drinking would be enjoyable, enhancing their leisure and their lives. Smaller proportions also indicated that they expected that their drinking would inflict negative consequences. These predictably included nausea and hangovers. They also included health damage and getting into trouble with the police. As Table 2.2 shows, girls reported expecting slightly higher levels of most negative consequences than did the boys.

Young women and alcohol

'I Don't Wanna Be A Boy, I Wanna Be
A Girl! I Wanna Do Things That'll
Make Ya
Hair Curl! ...
...Yeah! And Act Like A Child And Act
Like A Child!
If It Sutes Me Cause We've Got Cause
She's Got Girl Power,
We Glower Coming Home Drunk In
The Midnight Hour Girl......'

(Shampoo 1996)

'I'm going out tonight–I'm feelin' alright
Gonna let it all hang out
Wanna make some noise—really raise my voice
Yeah, I wanna scream and shout.
No inhibitions–make no conditions
Get a little outta line
I ain't gonna act politically correct
I only wanna have a good time.
The best thing about being a woman
Is the prerogative to have a little fun . . .'

(Shania Twain 1998)

As the lyrics from these two popular songs indicate, many western women have come a long way from when they were expected to be shy, dignified, and retiring. Even so, it would seem that 'ladette culture' (an expression derived from 'Jack the Lad,' meaning a male amiable 'rogue' who behaves in a noisy, riotous way) may be more of a feature of the UK than elsewhere. The reasons for this are unclear, although a number of theories have been suggested. These include the possibility that young women in the UK have more social freedom than those in some other countries and the possibility that alcohol advertising has been especially targeted at young women.

This issue of women and power was shown in a study by Barnes-Powell (1997). The study showed that for these young women their drinking patterns were closely linked to their daily lives and what they perceived as their place in society. Drinking alcohol was viewed as positive. It was symbolic of the opportunities to try new and varied experiences. The effects of alcohol were generally described as good, positive feelings. However, an interesting aspect was their view of alcohol from quite early in their lives as liberating. These young women described alcohol as as a 'mood setter', a 'confidence booster', and a 'disinhibitor'. It enabled them to feel powerful and to express themselves. Importantly they described becoming drunk as 'time out' from real life. The feelings when drunk were exciting and different from their normal lives, which they described as having little control over and generally not containing much pleasure. Not all the young women in Barnes-Powell's study drank in this way, but those who did not conformed in many ways to the more traditional behaviour of women.

It is not so long ago that some bars in Britain and elsewhere discriminated against women by refusing them entry (Lupton 1979). Those days, fortunately, have gone thanks to social changes and anti-sex discrimination legislation. Some British bars and clubs now discriminate in favour of women by offering them cheaper entry or drink prices than are available for men. It appears from several studies that heavy drinking among young adult women has been increasing rapidly since the late 1990s. The latest finding, that teenage girls out-binge the boys, is remarkable. It remains to be seen whether this is purely a temporary phenomenon, or the beginning of a longer-term change in drinking patterns. The UK's high level of binge drinking among teenage girls is very unusual. In the great majority of other countries surveyed (32 out of 35) binge drinking remained more common among boys than among girls. Something interesting has been happening with women's drinking in the UK, Ireland, and the Isle of Man. This is considered further below.

These results add weight to the two previous ESPAD surveys, together with evidence from several other studies. These suggest that episodic heavy drinking, now often called 'binge drinking' is commonplace amongst young people and that the adverse effects associated with this behaviour such as hangovers, nausea, absenteeism, accidents, injuries, disorder, and interpersonal conflict are widespread. Moreover, rates of alcohol-related liver disease mortality are increasingly rapidly. Cases of alcohol-related liver disease, traditionally a condition of middle or old age, are even being noted among teenagers. Increasing numbers of young people are also being recorded who have alcohol-related psychiatric problems.

UK teenagers were also distinctive in relation to both the levels of problems they had experienced because of their drinking and their expectancies relating to alcohol consumption. These teenagers were particularly likely to report having experienced high levels of problems cause by alcohol. The UK ranked seventh in this respect, following Denmark, the Isle of Man, Finland, Lithuania, Ireland, and Latvia. Paradoxically, UK teenagers reported high levels of positive expectancies related to drinking, together with their peers from Finland, Ireland, and the Czech Republic. This finding has implications for the reasons why some young people drink heavily. As noted in some previous studies, most UK drinkers report enjoying their alcohol consumption, even if it sometimes harms them. Clearly, people drink for complex reasons and are strongly influenced by their companions and by social pressure. This fact probably explains why most past attempts to modify the drinking habits of young people, through educational programmes and campaigns, have failed to achieve their goals. Alcohol education is discussed in more detail in Chapter 7. It does not have an impressive track record.

Alcohol and other drugs

It has been clear for a long time that heavy drinkers are often also smokers and users of illicit drugs (M. A. Plant and M. L. Plant 1992). The level of tobacco smoking in the UK has declined as it has in many other developed countries.

Even so, 26 per cent of adults smoke, especially those with less education and in lower income groups (Office of National Statistics 2005). Young people in the UK report high levels of experience with illicit drugs, especially cannabis. There is a similar picture in Ireland and the Isle of Man (M. A. Plant and M. L. Plant 1992, Hibell *et al.* 2004).

There is no doubt that the club scene that has developed in Britain has done much to popularise the use of illicit drugs such as cocaine, ecstasy (MDMA), and Special K (ketamine). As noted by Thornton (1996):

> 'Alcohol is the most widely used intoxicant of club cultures, if only because it is legal, easily available and inexpensive... Research has shown that many clubbers are often polydrug users who tend to abstain from drugs other than marihuana outside clubs and raves.' (p21).

The most frantic pubbing and clubbing occur on Friday and Saturday nights. It has long been evident that the speed of weekend drinking is often faster than that occurring during the week (Mass Observation 1943 p.171). Sunday, for many young clubbers, is recovery time. Youthful heavy drinking and illicit drug use involve people from all walks of life. Most want to be fit for school/college/work on Monday, even though some fail to manage this (Parker *et al.* 1998, Parker and Egginton 2002, Egginton *et al.* 2002).

Alcohol and the family

Previous ESPAD findings showed that teenagers who drink heavily and with problems are particularly likely to use illicit drugs, to smoke, and to come from single parent families. In the UK, the latter are at high risk of being on low incomes and headed by an adult who is unemployed. ESPAD included a question in 1999 asking teenagers if their parents usually know where they were on a Saturday night. In 2003 teenagers were asked if their parents know where they were in the evenings. The 1999 survey showed that many UK teenagers (51 per cent) reported that their parents did not always know where they were on Saturday night. This was a much higher proportion than in some other countries, such as Cyprus, Denmark, France, Hungary, Malta, and Portugal (Hibell *et al.* 2001). These findings suggest that UK parents are much less likely than parents in some other countries to monitor the whereabouts of their teenage sons and daughters. This fact coincides with the much heavier drinking reported by UK teenagers in comparison with those in some other countries where parents are more inclined to monitor their children's leisure activities.

Heavy teenage drinking is widespread across the social spectrum. Even so, the heavy use of both alcohol, cigarettes, and illicit drugs is particularly commonplace amongst teenagers from single parent households and from families in which parents do not set rules about their behaviour (Miller 1997, Miller and Plant 1999).

A series of surveys of the drinking habits of 11–15-year-old school students in England has been carried out for the Department of Health. This has shown that there has been a considerable increase in alcohol consumption amongst such young people since 1990:

> 'The average weekly consumption among pupils who drank in the last 7 days increased from 5.3 units in 1990 to 9.9 units in 1998, and has fluctuated around this figure since then, showing no clear pattern. In 2004, the average weekly consumption among pupils who drank was 10.7 units. In contrast to previous years, the average weekly consumption of alcohol by girls who drank was at a similar level to that of boys. Among those who drank, girls drank an average of 10.2 units in the previous 7 days in 2004, compared with 11.3 units among boys.'

These findings are shown in Figs 2.5 and 2.6.

Alcohol consumption levels have also risen amongst Scottish school students aged 13 and 15 years. The increase over the period 1994–2004 is shown in Fig. 2.7.

There are regional variations in drinking patterns. There are predictably more abstainers among young Muslims than in the general population. In addition, there are large minorities of teenagers in the Western Isles of

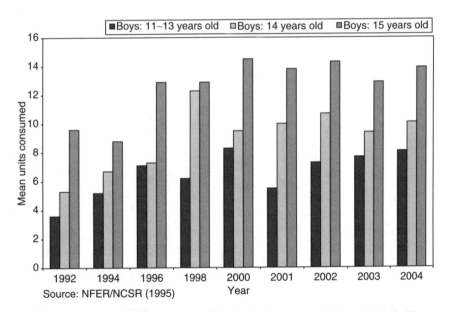

Fig. 2.5 English boys' mean consumption of alcohol in the past week (units, drinkers only) (1999–2004)

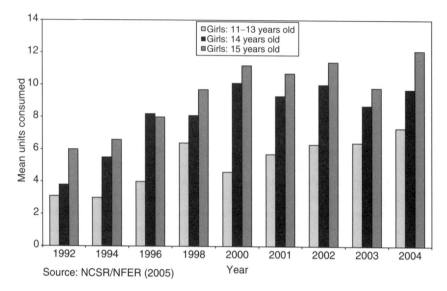

Fig. 2.6 English girls' mean consumption of alcohol in the past week (units, drinkers only) (1992–2004)

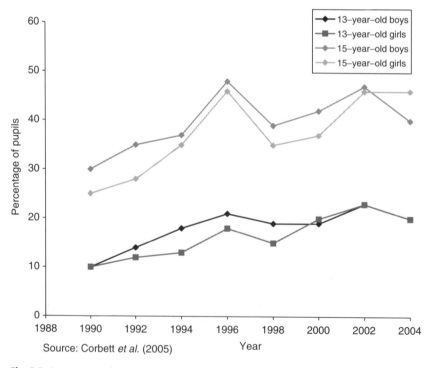

Fig. 2.7 Percentage of pupils aged 13 and 15 years who reported that they drank alcohol in the past week (Scotland) (1990–2004)

Scotland and in Northern Ireland who do not drink (Loretto 1994, Anderson and Plant 1996, Miller and M. A. Plant 2001b).

Loretto (1994 p.143), investigating drinking amongst 11–12 and 14–16-year-olds in Northern Ireland and Scotland, concluded that 'Northern Irish teenagers were less likely than their counterparts in the Scottish study group to have consumed an alcoholic drink.'

The 1999 ESPAD survey permitted a separate examination of drinking among school students aged 15 and 16 in Northern Ireland. This revealed that although 91% of boys and 68% of girls had consumed alcohol, teenage drinking was less commonplace than in the UK as a whole. In spite of this there were some reasons for concern. The proportion of boys drinking five or more drinks in a row in the past 30 days had risen since the 1995 ESPAD survey to reach 61%. This was higher than in other parts of the UK. In addition, roughly a fifth of girls and boys in Northern Ireland reported having last consumed alcohol at least partly in an open space such as a park, street, or school playground. Such settings involve more risks than drinking at home would do (Miller and M. A. Plant 2001b). The factual knowledge of teenagers about alcohol was poor.

Drinking by women

Approximately 90% of the women in Britain drink alcoholic beverages at least occasionally (M.L. Plant 1997, M.A. Plant and Cameron 2000, Academy of Medical Sciences 2004, Cabinet Office Prime Ministers' Strategy Unit 2004). During the last few years it has become evident that there has been an unprecedented rise in heavy drinking among young British women. A survey in 2000 showed that 8% of women aged 18–24 years had consumed at least 35 units of alcohol (more than a bottle of spirits) during the previous week. This was one of the first reports indicating that something remarkable was happening to young British women's drinking (M. L. Plant and M. A. Plant 2001, M. L. Plant et al. 2002a). This level of consumption is widely accepted as being 'high risk' in relation to possible adverse effects. A high level of heavy drinking among young women has subsequently been reported by other investigators (e.g. Office for National Statistics 2004, Williamson et al. 2003, M. A. Plant and M. L. Plant 2004, M. A. Plant et al. in 2005). This change mirrors that amongst teenage girls which has been described above.

Invaluable information about the nation's drinking has been collected by the General Household Survey (GHS). This routinely surveys a large sample of adults about a range of topics. The GHS has shown that between 1988 and 2000 the proportion of British males aged 16 and over drinking 36 units or more per week remained fairly stable at between 12–14%. In contrast the proportion of women who drank 15 units or more rose from 10–17%. The rise in drinking more than recommended 'low risk' amounts of alcohol during this period was most pronounced among women and men aged 16–24 years. Among young women the proportion drinking over 14 units per week more than doubled. It rose from 15 to 33%. Among young men the proportion drinking over 21 units rose from 31 to 41%. The proportion of young women who had consumed more than 35 units per week (defined as risky) rose from 3 to 9%. The proportions of young men who drank more than 50 units (defined as risky) increased from 10 to 14% (Walker *et al.* 2001).

Between 2000 and 2003 some measures of adult alcohol consumption remained relatively stable according to the GHS. Amongst British men the proportion who had consumed more than 8 units in one day fluctuated between 21–23%. Among women the proportion who had consumed more than 6 units in a day fell from 10% in 2000, 2001.

Frequent drinking is more commonplace among men and women on higher incomes. Amongst those earning at least £800 per week, 23% of women and 34% of men drank on five or more days. Only 10% of women and 18% of men earning up to £200 per week had done so. Men who were higher earners were more likely than lower earners to have consumed more than 8 units on at least one day. In contrast, women who were high earners were less likely to have consumed more than 6 units on at least one day. This is shown in Table 2.3.

Between 1998 and 2003 the proportions of women and men drinking in the past week remained stable or only changed slightly (women 59–60%; men 75%). The proportions of all adults drinking on five or more days in the last week remained fairly stable (13% women; 22–23% men). Even so the proportion of young women aged 16–24 who had done so fell from 7–8% between 1998 and 2002 to only 4% in 2003. There were some changes in the proportions of people drinking over 6 units (women) or 8 units (men) on at least one

Table 2.3 Percentage of people drinking more than 6–8 units on at least one day in the last week and usual gross weekly earnings

Income	Up to £200	£200.01 –£300	£300.01 –£400	£400.01 –£600	£600.01 –£800	£800.0 1 or more	Total
% Women	17	16	17	15	11	14	15
% Men	26	31	31	31	27	28	29

(Office of National Statistics Online, 2005).

Table 2.4 Percentage of women drinking more than 6 units on at least one day in last week and age

Age	1998	2000	2001	2002	2003
16–24	24	27	27	28	26
25–44	11	13	14	13	13
45–64	5	5	5	5	5
65 and over	1	1	1	1	1
Total	8	10	10	10	9

(Office of National Statistics Online, 2005).

Table 2.5 Percentage of men drinking more than 8 units on at least one day in last week and age

Age	1998	2000	2001	2002	2003
16–24	39	37	37	35	37
25–44	29	27	30	28	30
45–64	17	17	17	18	20
65 and over	4	5	5	5	6
Total	22	21	22	21	23

(Office of National Statistics Online, 2005).

day in the past week. These were a little higher in 2003 than they had been in 1998 as shown in Tables 2.4 and 2.5.

A survey of 6589 young people aged 11–15 years was carried out in Northern Ireland in 1997/98. This showed that 74% of those surveyed had consumed alcoholic drinks at some time. Amongst the youngest students only 5.6% of boys and 4.3% of girls reported monthly drinking and almost the same proportions reported weekly drinking. Amongst the oldest students more than 20% reported monthly drinking, while 44% of boys and 40% of girls reported weekly drinking. Amongst the boys who were drinking regularly, 31% had been drunk more than ten times. The corresponding proportion among girls was 23% (Health Promotion Agency for Northern Ireland 2000).

The term 'binge drinking' has been very widely used in the recent discussion about heavy and problematic alcoholic consumption in Britain. As explained in the Introduction to this book, until recently, the established meaning of this term was a prolonged session of two days or more during which other, normal activities were abandoned. During the last few years the term 'binge' has been increasingly used to mean drinking a lot in a single session. The Department of Health (1999) defined a 'binge' as consuming more than eight units for men and more than six units for women on at least one day per week. The Prime Minister's Strategy Unit (2003) defined a 'binge' as drinking over twice the recommended daily guidelines for daily drinking. This is six or more 'units' for females. The Strategy Unit concluded that there were 5,900,000 'binge drinkers' in Britain. People aged 16–24 years were those most likely to binge.

Williamson *et al.* (2003) have reported 38% of women in their twenties had engaged in 'binge drinking,' defined as consuming six or more units on at least one day in the week. The General Household Survey (GHS) for 2003 has shown that the proportion of women aged 16–24 years who had consumed six units or more on at least one day in the past week rose from 24% to 28% over the period 1998–2002. The GHS also indicated that women aged 16–24 were far more likely than others to have consumed this much. The most recent GHS indicated that 9% of all women aged 16 and above were 'heavy drinkers' in 2003. In that year 40% of women aged 16–24 had exceeded the daily benchmarks of alcohol on at least one day in the past week (Office of National Statistics 2004, 2005). The Parliamentary Office of Science and Technology (2005) has reported that '60% of alcohol consumed by women aged 20–29 is consumed in bouts of heavy drinking'. The recent upsurge in heavy drinking among young women has been remarkable. It may even escalate. The independent market analyst Datamonitor (2004) has predicted that alcohol consumption among young British women will increase by a further 31% over the next five years. The report suggested that the annual per capita alcohol consumption of young adult women will reach 291 litres. This report also noted: 'Young women's consumption in the UK is the highest in Europe and three times as large as the consumption in France and Italy'.

Mintel reported during August 2005 that alcohol consumption in Britain had increased by 5% during the past five years (Carvel 2005a).

Why are women drinking more?

Traditionally women have generally consumed much less alcohol than men (e.g. Dight 1976, Wilson 1980). Moreover, it has long been regarded as unacceptable for women to visit bars on their own, to drink heavily or to become intoxicated, especially in public. It has also been assumed that the presence of women in drinking situations acts as a restraining factor and keeps male drinkers in line. Things have clearly changed, at least in the UK. It is apparent that this double standard has been eroded and that large numbers of young women now believe that it is quite acceptable to drink heavily and to become conspicuously and often loudly drunk. This redefinition has been steady and rapid. It seems to have taken place among the most recent age group of young adult single women. Whether or not this is just a temporary blip or is the beginning of a profound and lasting social change cannot yet be determined. Even so, it is likely that this profound transformation will be a long-term one. The suggested reasons for this 'genderquake' (to use a term coined by Wilkinson 1994) include women's greater 'emancipation', including higher incomes, legal and political power and social freedom and the alleged special targeting of young women by alcohol advertising campaigns. It is certainly true that wine sales have risen considerably in recent years, while those of beer and spirits have not. Blackman (1998) has concluded that young British women now view the pub in a positive light.

Clearly some form of social change has been occurring in the UK that has not been evident elsewhere in Europe or elsewhere in the world to the same extent. In most other European countries girls and young women still drink much less than males (Bloomfield *et al.* 2005). There may be many suggested reasons for the increase in young women's drinking in the UK. These include the greater economic, political and social empowerment of UK women. In fact a review of women's empowerment has shown that UK women were ranked eighth out of 58 in countries that were considered. The seven countries in which women were classified as being more empowered than in the UK were Sweden, Norway, Iceland, Denmark, Finland, New Zealand and Canada. It does not appear that young women in these nations are drinking as much as young men even though in Finland and Norway the difference was not a big one. Moreover, Ireland was ranked sixteenth for women's empowerment even though their teenage girls have recently been drinking as much as teenage boys. This would suggest that the recent drinking habits of young women in the UK and Ireland have been influenced by additional factors (Lopez-Claros and Zahidi 2005).

It is notable that a lot of advertising has been targeted at young women. The effects of this have been reinforced by special cheap drinks offers for women in pubs and clubs, women's greater spending power and social assertiveness. One thing is clear. The traditional stigma that inhibited women from drinking heavily and being intoxicated in public has faded. 'Ladette culture' has re-defined heavy drinking as not only acceptable, but even desirable. This is conspicuous in most town and city centres during the evenings. This type of behaviour has been reported and sensationalized in numerous television programmes about, for example, Ibiza and 'Booze Britain.'

A perceptive insight into what has been happening has been provided by the work on changing urban nightlife by Chatterton and Hollands (2003). These authors have concluded that a number of features of Britain's newly developed night-time economy have influenced drinking by young women. They argue that the concentrations of newly corporatised drinking venues such as gentrified 'café-bars and hybrid bar/clubs' attract mainly young people who are more likely than older people to drink heavily. They maintain that the nightlife industry has especially targeted 'young, single and professional women'. They add:

> 'The 'equality' that many young women have gained in the nightlife sphere has often been on male terms, and contains their own negative consequences like increased levels of drunkenness, violence and drug consumption... The impact young women have had on transforming the character and atmosphere of urban nightlife is huge. This is particularly the case when one considers the limited role women played in the traditional pub (Hey 1986) and historically in the city in general (Wilson 1991). Much has changed even in the last decade, when Lees (1993) wrote: 'the pub is a male environment where girls may go with their boyfriend but do not feel confident to go on their own even in a group of girls'... numerous commentators have noted the powerful influence young female consumers are having on the transformation of nightlife premises and cultures of cities' (Barnard 1999, Wilkinson 1994, Hollands 1995, Andersson 2002).' (pp.148–9)

Chatterton and Hollands add that the increased economic activity of young women has fostered increased leisure spending and heavier drinking at least by those who have the incomes to permit it. There is no doubt that both teenage girls and young women are drinking more and that the adverse consequences of this are escalating. More research is needed to find exactly why this is happening. Moreover, it is as yet unknown if the recent changes in women's drinking will be lasting, or are just a temporary oddity. The important work of Chatterton and Hollands suggests that the conditions to maintain heavy drinking by young women and young men have now become set in durable brick, concrete, and stone. Many questions remain to be answered. It is unlikely that the advent of extended licensing hours in England and Wales will improve this serious situation.

Why do some people drink heavily?

As already noted, there are many reasons why people drink. Most of these are positive reasons, such as enjoyment of the taste and 'disinhibiting' effects of alcoholic drinks and to be sociable. This does not explain why people drink risky or obviously damaging quantities of alcohol. A recent study of British adults confirmed that most people enjoy their drinking and regard it as being 'a good thing' even if it clearly causes them problems (M. L. Plant et al. 2002b). A perceptive American commentator, David Elkind, has suggested that people, especially children and teenagers, believe that they are immortal and invulnerable so that they can engage in risky behaviour without any harm coming to themselves. Elkind (1967, 1984) has called this belief the 'Personal Fable'. This may at least partly explain why some individuals drink more than is wise in spite of numerous warnings and exhortations about possible dangers. A recent study of Belgian teenagers found that boys were more likely than girls to regard themselves as 'invulnerable' and 'omnipotent' (Goossens *et al.* 2002).

As noted previously, the Prime Minister's Cabinet Office (2004) reported that 5.9 million people in the UK were 'binge' drinkers and a further 1.8 million people were 'chronic' drinkers. The report also concluded that:

'Around a quarter of the population drink above former weekly guidelines and some 6 million above recommended daily guidelines'. The Government's recommended 'sensible weekly alcohol consumption guidelines' are up to 28 units of alcohol for a man and up to 21 units for a women. The maximum recommended daily limits are 2–3 units for a woman and 3–4 units for a man. It is recommended that people should have at least one alcohol-free day each week.'

There are wide variations between both levels of alcohol consumption and patterns of drinking in different countries. The variation in levels of per capita alcohol consumption (in litres of pure alcohol) is indicated by Table 2.6.

Table 2.6 Alcohol consumption (litres of pure alcohol) per head in 42 countries

| Country | Litres per head of 100% alcohol | | | | | |
	1970	1980	1990	2000	2001	2002
Austria	10.3	11.0	11.9	10.9	10.2	10.4
Belgium & Luxembourg (a)	9.0	10.9	11.1	9.0	9.2	9.3
Denmark	6.8	9.3	9.8	9.5	9.4	9.3
Finland	4.3	6.1	7.8	6.4	6.6	6.6
France	17.2	15.6	12.6	10.9	11.0	11.9
Germany (b)	12	13.3	12.3	10.7	10.7	10.6
Greece	–	–	7.5	6.9	7.0	7.1
Ireland, Rep of	5.9	7.4	7.3	9.9	10.1	10.2
Italy	16.0	13.9	9.5	8.0	7.8	7.8
Netherlands	5.5	8.6	8.1	8.1	8.0	7.9
Portugal	9.8	10.8	9.9	11.0	10.7	10.1
Spain	12.0	13.5	10.8	9.4	9.6	9.2

(Contd.)

Table 2.6 (Contd.)

Country	Litres per head of 100% alcohol					
	1970	1980	1990	2000	2001	2002
Sweden	5.8	5.6	5.8	5.3	5.4	5.4
UK	5.3	7.3	7.6	7.7	7.9	8.2
The rest of Europe						
Bulgaria, Rep. of	6.7	8.7	9.4	–	–	–
Croatia, Rep. of				–	–	–
Czech Republic				12.2	12.1	12.4
Hungary	9.9	12.9	12.1	11.0	11.0	11.1
Norway	3.6	4.6	4.1	4.4	4.4	4.7
Poland	5.1	8.4	6.7	6.7	6.4	6.7
Romania	5.8	7.6	8.5	10.0	9.8	10.7
Russian Federation				8.6	9.0	9.4
Slovak Republic				9.3	9.5	9.6
Slovenia, Rep. of				–	–	–
Switzerland	10.8	11.1	11.4	9.6	9.6	9.4
Ukraine				–	–	–
Africa						
Nigeria	–	–	–	–	–	–
South Africa	3.0	3.8	5.1	4.5	4.3	4.2
Asia						
China	–	–	–	3.8	3.8	3.8
Japan (includes sake)	4.8	5.6	6.5	6.5	6.4	6.4
Korea, Rep. of (beer only)	–	–	1.2	1.4	1.5	1.5
Philippines	–	4.0	–	–	–	–
Australasia						
Australia	7.8	9.4	8.4	7.6	7.9	7.9
New Zealand	6.3	8.2	7.9	6.9	7.0	7.2
North America						
Canada	6.4	8.7	7.3	6.5	6.6	6.8
USA	7.0	8.1	7.4	6.6	6.7	6.7
Central and South America						
Argentina (beer & wine)	11.8	9.5	7.2	5.9	5.8	6.0

Table 2.6 (Contd.)

Litres per head of 100% alcohol						
Country	1970	1980	1990	2000	2001	2002
Brazil (beer & wine)	0.7	1.3	2.5	2.7	2.7	2.6
Chile (beer only) (c)	5.6	6.4	4.5	1.2	1.2	1.1
Colombia (beer only)	1.4	1.8	2.5	1.3	1.2	1.2
Cuba (beer only)	0.8	1.2	1.5	1.0	1.0	0.3
Mexico (beer only) (c)	1.2	1.6	1.9	2.0	2.0	2.0
Peru (beer only) (c)	1.0	1.6	1.4	1.0	1.0	1.1
Venezuela (beer only) (c)	2.6	3.8	3.4	4.2	4.1	4.0

(a) Luxembourg has not been listed separately as cross border trading can lead to inaccuracies.
(b) Prior to 1991 data are for the Federal Republic of Germany only.
(c) Prior to 1991 beer and wine.
These figures include beer, wine and spirits and exclude cider, coolers, and FABs. Other countries; wine= 12% abv, beer= average strength, otherwise 5% abv for full strength and 0.5% abv for low alcohol.
(Source: British Beer and Pub Association 2004 p.93)

As this table shows, trends in per capita alcohol consumption over the period 1970–2002 have varied considerably. In some countries such as France and Italy consumption levels have fallen considerably. In others such as the UK and Ireland, they have risen.

There are clearly big differences in drinking cultures. Drunkenness is far more acceptable in some countries (e.g. the UK and Ireland) than it is in others (e.g. Cyprus, Italy, and Portugal) (MacAndrew and Edgerton 1969, Pittman and Raskin-White 1991). Another factor that varies between different countries is the way in which being drunk is perceived in practical terms. One small study showed that English, Dutch, and Swedish people had many words referring to being drunk as a behaviour. In contrast the Scots and the Greeks used more psychological definitions, meaning that becoming drunk involved entering an altered mental state. These results are hard to interpret. In spite of this they do add to the impression that drinking cultures are deeply rooted and powerful (Cameron *et al.* 2000).

The UK Strategy Unit further concluded that, applying the 6–8 units per day definition to the 2001 General Household Survey of Britain (England, Wales, and Scotland, N=20 149), it appeared that 5.9 million adult drinkers in Britain, or 15% of all adults, are classified as being 'binge drinkers.' The Strategy Unit further concluded (p.20) that those aged 16–24 years were most likely to be binge drinkers:

'Only a quarter of women of this age and around one in six men report never drinking more than 6–8 units per day. For some people, this type of drinking behaviour continues to middle age, with around one in three men and one in five women drinking twice the recommended daily benchmarks at least once a week between the ages of 45 and 64.'

Adults in Northern Ireland are more likely to abstain from drinking than their counterparts in most areas of England, Scotland, and Wales. Even so, 75% of Northern Irish men and 67% of women do drink. A recent survey showed that those people aged 44 years or below were more likely to drink than were those aged 45 and above. Adults from higher income households were more likely to drink than those from lower income groups. Drinkers were also more likely to be better educated and to have higher incomes than abstainers. This study examined the proportions of men and women who were 'binge drinkers'. The latter were defined as men who had consumed 10 units of alcohol on one session or women who had consumed 7 units in a session. The results of this analysis are shown in Table 2.7.

Table 2.7 Binge drinking amongst adults in Northern Ireland

Age	Men %	Women %
18–29	72	57
30–44	54	38
45–59	39	27
60–75	19	4

'Binge drinking' defined as drinking 10 units of alcohol in one session for men and 7 units for women. (Health Promotion Agency for Northern Ireland undated b, p.37)

As this table shows, younger adults were far more likely than older individuals to have consumed relatively large amounts of alcohol during a single session. 'Binge drinking', as defined in the previous paragraph, was most commonplace amongst semi-skilled and unskilled manual workers. It was least common amongst professional and intermediate non-manual workers. This study showed that amongst men, the most common location for binge drinking had been the pub (reported by 63%). In contrast, among women this had been their own home (51%) (Health Promotion Agency for Northern Ireland 2002).

The findings of a survey commissioned by BUPA Wellness were released in late October 2005. This found that almost a third of men and a fifth of women were drinking at least twice the recommended daily limits of 2–3 drinks for women and 3–4 drinks for men. This indicated that 11 million people in Britain were drinking in a risky way. A sixth of those surveyed reported that the expected new, extended bar opening hours would encourage them to drink more (Hope 2005).

Home drinking

There has been a trend for some time towards drinking at home. Recently a number of researchers have noted that many young adults drink at home before going out with friends. This phenomenon has been called 'pre-drinking'. The reasons that young people give for this behaviour include the fact that it saves money and that they wish to be at least mellow or drunk before joining their companions for a night clubbing and pubbing.

During August 2005 a report by the Department of the Environment noted that in the past decade expenditure on alcohol drunk at home had increased by 50% and that during the past year alcohol sales had risen by a remarkable 10%. In November 2005 the results of a survey were published. This showed that drinking in pubs and clubs had been declining for some years:

> 'Research agency TGI says in 1987, 17% of adults went out to drink more than once a week compared with the present figure of 12%, or 5.5 million adults. However, the number of people who drink has remained constant at 40 million.'

The survey says more people drink at home, with increased social stigma about drink driving one of the factors. Other figures show the number of 18–24-year-olds who visit the pub once a week has dropped. In 1987, this age bracket accounted for 18% of all those who went to the 'local' once a week, compared with 11% today. TGI director Julian Tooke said:

> 'There are likely to be many factors behind why pub going has steadily fallen in the last 15 years... Increased social stigma against drink driving and an increase in the number of people whose faith precludes them from drinking alcohol, are two factors which have no doubt played some part... The fact that pub-going figures are falling amongst the young, who are the main frequenters and the future of the market, bodes poorly for pubs. Fewer young people are drinking alcohol than 15 years ago. Ten million 18-to-30-year-olds drank then compared to only eight million today.'

The number of young people drinking in nightclubs has also dropped from 4 million in 2002 to 3 million today. And more women visit the pub—the gender split has changed from 64% men and 36% women in 1987 to 58% men and 42% women today. (BBC News Online November 2005a)

The monster in the middle: (what have we done to our town and city centres?)

> 'Police say harbourside nightclub Evolution is the worst trouble spot in the city for alcohol-fuelled violence. The force went to court yesterday to try to shut the club—only for its action to be halted on a technicality... During that time

(16 months) they say they were called to deal with 63 assaults, 40 incidents of disorder and nearly 200 other crimes, either inside or outside the Canon's Road club... One of the police officers involved in the case against the club, Superintendent Tim Lee, said: 'Evolution is identified as the number one problem in Bristol for alcohol-related violence on Friday and Saturday nights. There is a problem with alcohol-fuelled behaviour because of the nature of the premises. The younger age group who use the club become intoxicated and cause all sorts of incidents of crime.... Alcohol-fuelled assaults seem to be a consequence of the managements pack 'em and stack type of enterprise, having little regard for people's safety.' (Mathias 2005)

Some politicians have proclaimed the objective of converting the British people from being a nation that is notorious for getting drunk to a nation that drinks in a sedate 'continental' manner. This laudable objective has been severely undermined by what has been happening on the ground. During past decades most towns and cities have been developed to counter the movement of people away from central areas to live and shop out in the suburbs. Many urban centres have been regenerated and developed to establish leisure strips or entertainment areas. Many of these are now flourishing economically and attract large numbers of people. These areas, their patrons, and the jobs they create, have been described as the 'night time economy' (Hobbs 2002, Light 2005b). These areas have been designed to cater for large numbers of young adults out to have a good time. They typically contain concentrations of late-night drinking establishments (both pubs and clubs) some of which are enormous with room for over 1000 or more patrons. In some of these, known as 'maximum volume vertical drinking bars' most of those present drink while standing and many are quickly and frequently served with alcohol in bottles in settings that are so noisy and large that they have an anonymous atmosphere. The noise level is often deafening, many patrons are drunk and most are in their 20s and 30s. This presents a picture that is totally alien to people from countries such as France where public drinking usually occurs in small, relatively intimate establishments where most people sit and many drink while they enjoy a meal. The British will never evolve into well-behaved café-style drinkers in huge anonymised vertical drinking bars. Some of the owners of such premises would probably hate it if they did. They make far more money from selling alcohol than they do from selling food. Nottinghamshire's Chief Constable, Steve Green, has recently suggested that if the government wants a continental style of café culture they should 'build cafes' (Slack 2005a). As Chatterton and Hollands (2003) have commented, the newly developed 'urban nightscapes' feature a high proportion of pubs and clubs run by large national and international organizations such as Scottish and Newcastle and Bass and so-called 'pubcos' such as J.D. Wetherspoon. In their study of Bristol, Newcastle, and Leeds, they found over 60% of licensed premises to be under such ownership. Some of these agencies have heavily discounted alcohol prices. Many traditional male-oriented bars have been replaced by more sophisticated female-friendly establishments such as theme bars. Even so, these still promote heavy drinking sexual aggression, and violence. Chatterton and Hollands note that:

> '...problems including anti-social behaviour, outbursts of violence, excessive and under-age alcohol consumption, urinating and vomiting in the streets remain, whatever the type of nightlife. Many police forces have been unprepared for the scale of growth of nightlife, and, compared to other large sports or music events, street nightlife receives relatively few resources...Private door security firms and door men (or bouncers) play a key role in such networks, who in general outnumber police by a ratio of ten to one.' (p.54)

A number of factors have been identified as being associated with intoxication and aggression in and around bars. These are discussed in Chapter 7. It should be noted that the advent of the long bar in many pubs in the nineteenth century reportedly facilitated 'vertical' or 'perpendicular' drinking. This was considered to have been a negative development by Frederick Hackwood, who commented that patrons could be served more rapidly if they were standing (Hackwood 1910). It has also been suggested that the modern, large urban bar type of development has served to marginalise some young people because they cannot fully participate in this lifestyle. It is also possible that the anonymity of the large town pub fosters more extreme behaviours (such as heavy drinking) than would be evident in a smaller, local pub. (Hollands and Chatterton 2001, Chatterton and Hollands 2003). There is evidence, for example, that density of bars and other licensed premises in an area is associated with increased levels of heavy drinking, drunkenness, violence, and other forms of crime (Colorado Alcohol and Drug Abuse Division 1990, Dilulio 1995, Scribner et al. 1995, Lipton and Gruenwald 2002). A Dutch study by Van Oers and Garretsen (1993) indicated that bar and off-licence density was associated with higher levels of local traffic injuries. Interestingly, Lipton and Gruenwald found that alcohol problems were not associated with the density of restaurants in an area. It has also been reported that intoxication is associated with the seating capacity of bars (Graham 1985). This evidence is borne out by the fact that many of Britain's leisure strips have become notorious for drunken disorder. One commentator described her local city centre as 'Animal Farm'. She added that nobody would go there unless they wanted to get drunk. A uniformed police officer informed one of the authors: 'I really hate Friday and Saturday nights. They ruin my job. Late night bars just get people pissed and violent'.

One vivid account of the ways in which some bars foster heavy drinking has been provided by Asthana (2005):

'8 p.m., Saturday. A woman in a red dress with plastic 'devil horns' swings her body in a circle, shrieking as she squirts whipped cream over her friends. Laughing, she clasps her hands round a pint of cider, lifts it to her lips and gulps down the contents.

It could be any weekend night, in any town or city. It is a scene replayed inside the enormous, barn-like bars that have become temples to drink. With a friend, Liz, I had travelled to Reading to test Britain's drinking culture. We were 40 miles from London, but we could have been anywhere.

We entered the bar and were hit by a wave of noise. The lack of tables made 'vertical drinking'—standing up, drink in hand and therefore drinking more—the norm as young people packed in, shouting to be heard over the loud music. On the wall, a list of football fixtures was just visible under a row of coloured lights.

Raucous groups of women were downing Bacardi Breezers, while men in checked shirts scoured for a 'pull'. This was one of many bars in town with a late licence and we were still drinking long after 11 p.m. Late-night drinking is already here in England and Wales and you don't have to look very far.

It seemed as though everyone was drunk, but no one was turned away from the bar. The bouncers walked straight past the woman with the whipped cream, the couple simulating sex in the corner and the two barmaids gyrating to Beyoncé's 'Crazy in Love'.

The punters were there for one reason; to get completely drunk, off their faces, tanked up, pissed—and the staff were not going to stop them. Over three and a half hours, my friend and I bought 12 rounds. Every 20 minutes on cue, we returned to the same part of the bar and the same barwoman and ordered drink after drink.

This is what we ordered: a bottle of wine; four bottles of a vodka-based alcopop; four vodka shots, each a different colour; two more bottles of vodka-based alcopops; three double sambucas; a double gin and tonic and a double vodka and tonic; three double tequilas; a second bottle of wine; four vodka alcopops; two double tequilas; two more double gin and tonics; two more double sambucas.

It totalled 64 units, 32 each. The barwoman recognized our faces and thought the drinks were for the two of us. But she never stopped serving—enough alcohol to kill each of us. We did not drink it all, but handed it on to customers in the bar. We had to.

We left at 11.30 p.m., the end of our typical night in a pub in England. People drinking until stupefied before spilling out into the street, fighting, shouting, drunk in the gutter. It was mayhem, fuelled by bar staff and a pub industry all too willing to serve drink after drink after drink. No questions asked.' (pp 8–9)

The fact that some bars serve huge quantities of alcohol to drinkers is indisputable. This fact has been borne out by police and media reports (e.g. Thompson 2005). Ironically, a number of other countries where alcohol consumption has traditionally been relatively sedate, even though heavy, appear to be developing a binge drinking culture even as their national alcohol consumption has been declining. It has for example, been reported that medical experts in Italy have warned that 'the opening of large numbers of pubs and late-night drinking establishments' has led to serious problems. It has been reported that 'lager louts' in Padua have caused so much disorder that 'authorities have virtually banned drinking in the town centre' (Johnston 2004).

Alcohol consumption and price

Alcohol consumption, like that of any consumer commodity, is influenced by price. During recent decades the proportion of household expenditure that has been spent on alcohol has fallen while alcohol consumption has risen. In other words, the affordabilty of alcohol has been increasing. This is elaborated in Fig. 2.8

As this figure shows, the per capita alcohol consumption of people aged 15 years and older in the UK rose from 6.3 litres of pure alcohol in 1964 to 11.5 litres in 2004. This is an increase of 83%. In contrast the percentage of

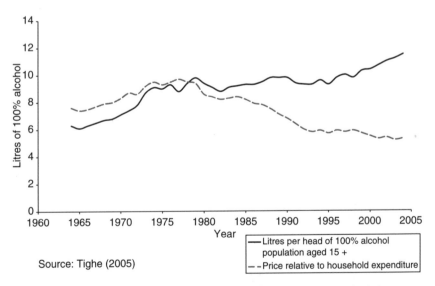

Source: Tighe (2005)

Fig. 2.8 Consumption of alcohol in the UK (per person aged 15 and over) relative to proportion of household incomes

household incomes spent on alcoholic beverages fell from 7.6% to 5.3%, a decrease of 30%. There is no doubt that a major factor (probably the greatest single one) for the increase in alcohol consumption in the UK has been the substantial rise in the affordability of drinking.

Trends in beverage preference

As indicated in the previous chapter, the British have traditionally mainly been beer drinkers. During the past forty years beer has lost its pre-eminence as other forms of alcoholic beverage have been adopted. In spite of this, beer is still by far the most popular drink in the United Kingdom. In 1964 a total of 71% of the alcohol consumed in the UK was in the form of beer, while spirits accounted for 18.3% and wine a mere 9%. In 2004 the proportion of alcohol consumed in the form of beer had dropped to only 44.5% while wine had increased its share to 27.7%. The proportion of alcohol consumed in the form of spirits had risen slightly to 19.8%. In fact beer and cider consumption actually rose during this period (from 94.2 litres per head to 109.3 litres per head). This growth was, however, far surpassed by the rise in wine drinking (from 3.1 litres per head in 1964 to 21.9 litres per head in 2004 plus an additional 4.9 litres in the form of wine-based coolers and flavoured alcoholic beverages (alcopops) (Tighe 2005). Alcopops include drinks such as Bacardi Breezer, Fusion, Glitz Ice, Hazy Dayz, Lovebyte, Pirhana, and WKD.

Chapter 3

The consequences of drinking: the good, the bad, and the ugly

'A teenager who was found dead in bed had downed three pints and 16 spirits in just 40 minutes.' (Disley 2005b).

'A British tourist died after downing a pint of mixed spirits during a holiday pub crawl.' (Alcohol Focus Scotland 2005).

Alarmed hospital staff say Perth's drinking problem is spiralling out of control as boozed-up revellers flood into the city's casualty wards every weekends.' (Alcoholics Anonymous Reviews 2005).

'Sherie Evans found out how high a price youngsters can pay for binge drinking when she fell from a wall and broke her neck.' (Pearlman 2005)

This chapter considers the positive and negative effects of drinking and reviews some of the evidence of changing trends in these consequences. As noted above, most people start to drink because of curiosity and a wish to join in a popular activity. Thereafter, as indicated in Table 2.1 in the previous chapter, most continue to drink because they enjoy the effects of alcoholic beverages. A recent survey of British adults showed that most people rated their drinking as being 'enjoyable' or 'very enjoyable'. Very few indicated that it was not. British teenagers typically report that they have positive expectancies of drinking. The same is true of teenagers in other countries with patterns of episodic heavy drinking. These include Ireland and Denmark (Hibell *et al.* 2004). Paradoxically, teenagers in countries where many young people report both heavy drinking and adverse effects are precisely those who also report having the most positive expectancies of drinking. Binge drinking is socially approved, esteemed, and eventful in the view of many teenagers. It brings both pleasure and pain. Sipping wine from a small glass during a family meal simply has a different meaning (or social construction). It is on a different level of experience, being far more low key. Some teenagers are, of course, able to do both. They sometimes share a meal-time drink with parents or other relatives, but also enjoy going out and getting drunk with their friends.

A little bit of what you fancy...

Most people drink because they enjoy doing so. Fortunately moderate alcohol consumption is not usually harmful and can even be beneficial to health. This fact means that alcohol does not have to be treated in exactly the same way as tobacco. The latter is simply damaging to health, so it is advisable not to smoke. Smoking kills approximately 120,000 people annually in the UK (Jarvis 2004).

Heavy drinkers are more likely to die young than are people who drink less. Abstainers also have relatively high rates of premature mortality. Some abstainers are 'sick quitters,' people who once drank heavily but who have stopped drinking. Other abstainers may not drink because they are in poor health, or have religious views that inhibit them from drinking. It is also possible that some abstainers have more restricted networks of social contacts than people who drink. There is evidence that moderate drinking is protective against both coronary heart disease and ischaemic stroke (stroke caused by a blood clot in the brain cutting off blood supply to the surrounding area) among middle aged and elderly men and women (e.g. Grønbæk *et al.* 1995, Stampfer *et al.* 1988, see M. L. Plant 1997 for review). It has at times been suggested that some beverages, such as red wine, are especially health enhancing. Grønbæk and colleagues, for example, concluded that moderate wine drinking reduced mortality, while moderate spirit drinking had the opposite effect. Studies in this field have produced mixed results. As previously summarized by M. L. Plant (1997 p.79):

The topic of beverage specificity has been addressed in other studies but the findings have been inconsistent. Some studies noted wine being most beneficial (St Leger *et al.* 1979, Renaud and De Logeril 1992, Klatsky and Armstrong 1993). Friedman and Kimball (1986) reported wine and beer more beneficial than spirits. Others found no difference by beverage type (Rosenberg *et al.* 1981, Klatsky *et al.*, 1986, Stampfer *et al.* 1988). In a review of beverage type and potential differences in protective effects, Rimm *et al.* (1996) noted:

'Results from observational studies, where alcohol consumption can be linked directly to an individual's risk of coronary heart disease, provide strong evidence that all alcoholic drinks are linked with lower risk. Thus a substantial proportion of the benefit is from alcohol rather than from other components of each type of drink.' (p.731)

The protective effect of moderate drinking on health is a tangible one. This has, for example, been demonstrated in Canada (Single *et al.* 1998) and the UK. A recent detailed study by Britton concluded that:

'At a population level in England and Wales current alcohol consumption marginally reduces mortality, but the favourable mortality balance is only found among older men and women. The contribution of alcohol-related deaths to overall mortality differs in countries in Europe. The risks associated with alcohol consumption are unlikely to be substantially different depending on the beverage type, but they are likely to be increased when alcohol is consumed in 'binges'. Additional deaths could be avoided if the population followed the UK government's 'sensible drinking' guidelines.' (Britton 2001 p.ii)

The merits of beginning to drink early in life and with family members are complex. This type of experience is more common in some countries such as France than it is in Britain. Even so, there is evidence suggesting that beginning to drink at an early age is associated with heavy drinking and alcohol problems in later life (Hingson and Kenkel 2004, York et al. 2004, Pitkänen et al. 2005). An analysis of UK survey findings from a study of 15 and 16-year-olds showed that fewer than a fifth reported that their parents had taught them to drink. Those who had been 'taught' came from generally better off families. They were more likely to be frequent drinkers than other teenagers, but also consumed less when they did drink (Miller and M. A. Plant 2005).

Like the two earlier ESPAD surveys, that of 2003 indicated that UK teenagers reported high levels of problems related to alcohol. Moreover, teenagers in the UK were some of those most likely to report having positive expectations about drinking. This was a characteristic of teenagers in countries where they also reported the highest rates of heavy drinking, together with both early and recent drunkenness. These countries included Finland, Ireland, the Czech Republic, the Isle of Man, and Denmark. This is elaborated in figures 3.1–3.4:

These findings support the conclusion that teenagers in countries where youthful heavy drinking is commonplace, accept adverse effects as part of the price to be paid for having a good time drinking to excess. The survey also showed that the opposite was evident in countries in which fewer teenagers drank heavily. These included Portugal and France. In countries like these teenagers had less positive expectancies and experienced far fewer problems. The prevalence of problems reported by UK teenagers is shown in Table 3.1

As this table shows, the most common problems were damage to objects or clothing and loss of money or valuables. Teenagers also reported problems related to accidents, injuries, relationships, and delinquency.

Evidence shows that, in general, whenever alcohol consumption rises or falls, levels of the problems associated with heavy drinking do the same. This is discussed in more detail in Chapter 7. There are exceptions to this tendency and some problems display rather different trends because other factors as well as alcohol may have an effect. The levels of alcohol-related problems that are recorded reflect not only how much people drink, but also the policies and

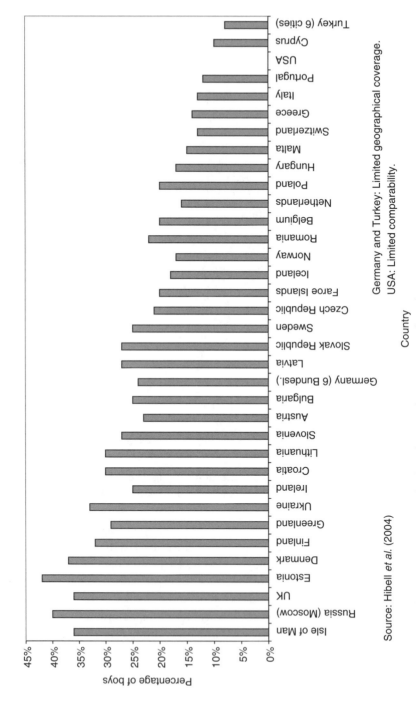

Source: Hibell *et al.* (2004)

Germany and Turkey: Limited geographical coverage.
USA: Limited comparability.

Fig. 3.1 Percentage of boys who have been drunk at the age of 13 or younger (2003)

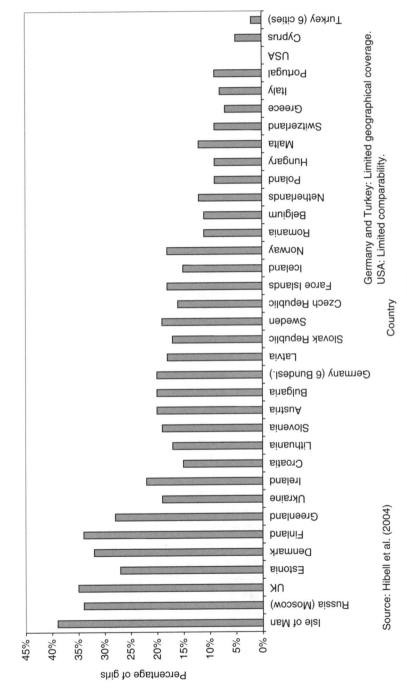

Fig. 3.2 Percentage of girls who have been drunk at the age of 13 or younger (2003)

Source: Hibell et al. (2004)

Germany and Turkey: Limited geographical coverage.
USA: Limited comparability.

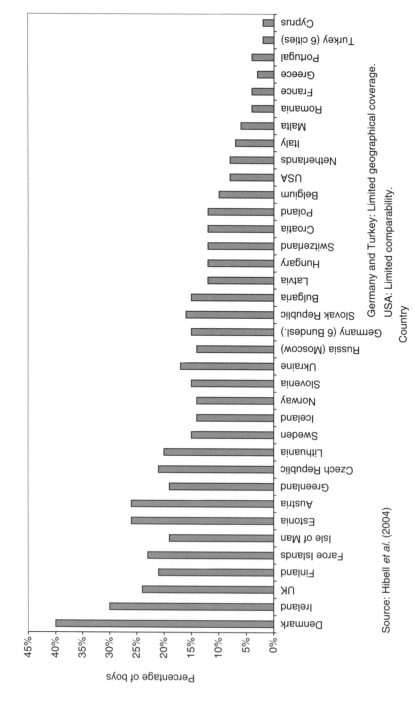

Fig. 3.3 Percentage of boys who have been drunk 10 times or more during the last 12 months (2003)

Source: Hibell *et al.* (2004)

Germany and Turkey: Limited geographical coverage.
USA: Limited comparability.

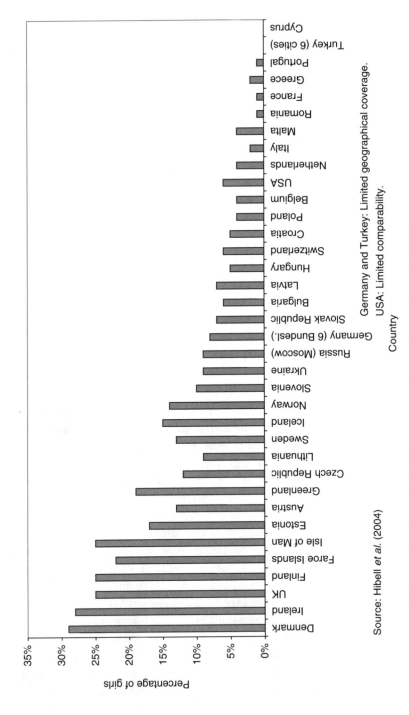

Fig. 3.4 Percentage of girls who have been drunk 10 times or more during the last 12 months (2003)

Source: Hibell *et al.* (2004)

Germany and Turkey: Limited geographical coverage.
USA: Limited comparability.

Table 3.1 UK teenagers' problems caused by own drinking

Type of problem	Boys (%)	Girls (%)
Engaged in sex you regretted next day	9	12
Engaged in unprotected sex	6	11
Scuffle or fight	12	11
Victimised by robbery or theft	2	2
Trouble with police	9	11
Performed poorly at school	3	4
Damage to objects or clothing	21	28
Loss of money or valuables	16	22
Accident or injury	14	17
Hospitalised or admitted to emergency room	2	3
Quarrel or argument	13	18
Problems in relationship with friends	8	11
Problems in relationships with parents	6	10
Problems in relationships with teachers	1	1

(Hibell et al. 2004)

methods of the agencies that collect this information. Some recording is better and more thorough than others. Although it is clear that most people are usually not adversely affected by their drinking, a substantial minority do report some form of negative consequences. A survey of British adults carried out in 2000 showed that many people reported experiencing consequences such as hangovers and 'memory loss' due to their drinking in the past year. Smaller numbers of men and women reported having experienced more serious problems. These were work/housework problems, marital/partner relationship problems, physical ill health, drunken driving, and fighting. This is shown in Figs. 3.5 and 3.6 (M. L. Plant *et al.* 2002b). It is clear that many people in Britain regard hangovers and their attendant discomfort as being acceptable 'battle damage', a price worth paying for their drinking sprees. Even people who have experienced many adverse effects from their drinking usually report that they still view their drinking as being enjoyable.

It is well-established that heavy drinking is associated with crime, including violence (Collins 1982, Plant M. A. *et al.* 2002). The study noted in the previous paragraph found that the experience of childhood and adult sexual abuse was associated with later heavy drinking, as well as alcohol and other problems in adulthood (M. L. Plant *et al.* 2004, M. L. Plant *et al.* 2005). In addition, aggression

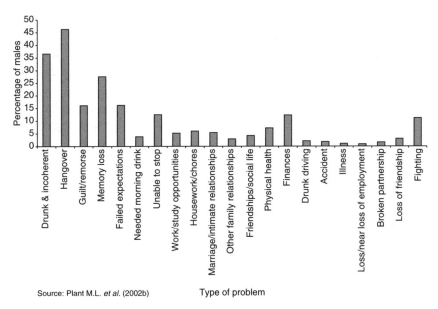

Source: Plant M.L. *et al.* (2002b)

Fig. 3.5 Alcohol problems reported in the past year amongst British male drinkers

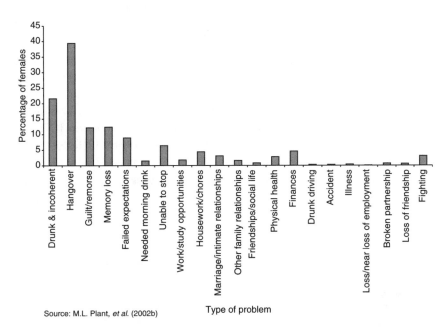

Source: M.L. Plant, *et al.* (2002b)

Fig. 3.6 Alcohol problems reported in the past year amongst British female drinkers

and violence by partners was associated with drinking by one or both of those involved. Drinking by an aggressive partner was associated with increased severity of the incident and increased fear (Graham *et al.* 2004). A study by Kaukinen (2002) reported that the victims of violence subsequently engaged in heavy episodic drinking and experienced negative alcohol-related consequences. This is also highlighted in dating violence and date rape (Rickert *et al.* 2002)

The Forensic Science Service (FSS) reported in September 2005 that 15% of rape victims recorded by the 2001 British Crime Survey reported having been raped when they were 'incapable of consent' due to alcohol consumption. In addition the FSS reported that most samples it receives that are related to drug-assisted rape involve a high level of alcohol, not illicit substances (Home Office Online 2005). A survey of public attitudes to rape by Amnesty International revealed that 30% of the British public believed that rape victims who had been drunk or flirtatious were at least partly responsible for being assaulted (Channel Four 2005). Prejudiced attitudes like this may explain why the UK has a shamefully low conviction rate in relation to the pitifully small proportion of rape cases that go to court. Another frightening development occurred in November 2005 when the front page headline in the Times read: 'Women can't claim rape when drunk, judge rules.' A High Court judge ruled in a rape case that 'drunken consent is still consent'. (Gibb *et al.* 2005). It seems the old equation of 'woman + alcohol = sex' now has a legal basis. Clearly young women who think they have equal rights with men are dangerously mistaken.

There is already evidence of an increase in the adverse health effects of heavy drinking among young British women. These include a significant rise in alcohol-related psychiatric morbidity among teenage girls (Aylin 2004) and even cases of alcohol-related liver disease among the same group (Gilmore 2004) and amongst young women in general (Department of Health 2001). Evidence suggests that heavy drinking is associated with many health problems (M. L. Plant 1997, Wilsnack and Wilsnack 1997). These include the following:

Accidents, injuries
Malnutrition and eating disorders
Anxiety and depression
Memory loss
Self-harm
Unprotected sex and unplanned pregnancy
Sexual and non-sexual assault
Alcohol poisoning
Liver-related morbidity and mortality
Fetal Alcohol Spectrum Disorder (FASD)
Cancer
Suicide.

It has recently been reported that there has been a 25% rise in cases of oral cancer in the past decade. This is associated with rising alcohol consumption (Meikle 2005). Heavy drinking during pregnancy poses risk of harm to the development of the fetus. In some cases this leads to permanent physical and psychological damage (Abel 1998, M. L. Plant *et al.* 1999). It is not known to what extent young women in general may be aware of this type of risk, or what their views are concerning what, if anything, they should drink when pregnant. Evidence suggests that heavy episodic drinking in the preconception time is associated with unintended pregnancy (Naimi *et al.* 2003). This subject has important implications for child health and future prevention policy.

A US study has indicated that:

> 'people who began binge drinking at the age of 13 years and continued to do so throughout adolescence were nearly 4 times as likely to be overweight or obese and almost 3.5 times as likely to have high blood pressure when they were 24 years old than were people who never or rarely drank heavily during adolescence.' (Oesterle *et al.* 2004).

Obesity is a growing health problem in the UK as in other Western countries. Evidence suggests an increased risk of weight gain in young women who drink heavily. Rising alcohol consumption among women may be adding to the problem of obesity in the population (Morgan 2004). It has been reported that alcohol consumption is associated with eating disorders (Wiederman and Pryor 1996, Morgan *et al.* 1999). There is some evidence (McCormack and Carman 1989) that the motivations for alcohol use and problem drinking are similar to those of eating disorders such as bulimia. Such motivations include stress reduction and mood alteration. These may also be linked with behaviours such as self-harm (Ystgaard *et al.* 2003, Spender 2004, Claes *et al.* 2005). Heavy drinking is associated with a constellation of other adverse consequences that are directly or indirectly related to health. These include experience of having drinks 'spiked', dangerous driving behaviour and having a large number of sexual partners (M. A. Plant and M. L. Plant 1992, M. L. Plant 1997). There is considerable evidence linking heavy drinking among young people with rape (Mohler-Kuo *et al.* 2004) and with presentation to Emergency Departments with acute alcohol intoxication (Woolfenden *et al.* 2002).

The Prime Ministers Cabinet Office (2004) reported that alcohol misuse cost the National Health Service £1.7 billion per year. It was also noted that £95 million was being spent on specialist alcohol treatment. The report acknowledged that there were over 30,000 annual hospital admissions for alcohol dependence and up to 20,000 premature deaths associated with alcohol. It was calculated that the cost of alcohol-related crime was £7.3 billion and that 360,000 incidents of domestic violence were alcohol-related. Other forms of harm that were acknowledged were as follows:

'1.2 million violent incidents (around half of all violent crimes); increased anti social behaviour and fear of crime—61% of the population perceive alcohol-related violence is worsening; up to 22,000 premature deaths per annum; at peak times, up to 79% of all admissions to accident and emergency departments; up to 1,000 suicides; up to 17 m working days lost through alcohol relayed absence; between 780,000 and 1.3m children affected by parental alcohol problems; Increased divorce—marriages where there are alcohol problems are twice as likely to end in divorce.' (p.7)

The report noted that:

'Binge drinkers and those who drink to get drunk are likely to be aged under 25. They are more likely to be men, although women's drinking has been rising fast over the last ten years. Binge drinkers are at increased risk of accidents and alcohol poisoning. Men in particular are more likely both to be a victim of violence and to commit violent offences. There can also be a greater risk of sexual assault. The impacts on society are visible in, for example, high levels of attendance at A&E related to alcohol. 5.9 million people have drunk more than twice the daily guidelines in the past week.' (pp 13–14)

Many recent studies have noted that heavy drinking has increased among teenagers (especially girls), young women and that rates of alcohol-related liver disease, psychiatric morbidity and alcohol-related violence have been increasing (e.g. M. A. Plant and Cameron 2000, M. A. Plant and M. L. Plant 2001, Plant et al. 2002. Hibell et al. 2004, M.A. Plant et al. 2005). As noted in the preceding chapter, the recent rise in heavy drinking by young women has attracted a lot of attention and concern. One reason for the latter has been suggestions that intoxicated women are increasingly being targeted as easy prey by rapists (Kirkham 2005). As noted in the previous chapter, many women visit bars and clubs. Research has suggested that they do this for 'companionship, diversion, and validation of oneself' (Parks et al. 1998). It has also been noted that many women seek a 'managed' level of intoxication—enough to enjoy alcohol's effects, but not enough to lose control (De Crespigny 2001). It is also clear that many women who frequent bars experience (mainly male) aggression and violence (Parks et al. 1998, De Crespigny 2001).

'Alcohol problems among young people have reached crisis proportions around the globe. Calculated from data published by the World Health Organization, in the year 2000, when people aged 15–29 years comprised 26% of the world's population, this age group lost more than 37% of the disability adjusted life years (DALYs). Worldwide, alcohol use in 2000 caused 285 000 deaths and loss of nearly 22 million DALYs among 15–29-year-olds.' (Jernigan and Mosher 2005)

Some national trends

Overall levels of alcohol-related mortality (from alcohol-related liver disease and other causes) have been rising steadily throughout Britain. As shown in Fig. 3.7 and 3.8, this rise has become more rapid since the mid 1990s.

In contrast the number of officially recorded drunkenness offenders in Britain has been declining. This is shown in Figs. 3.9 and 3.10. The fall has been especially dramatic in Scotland where drunkenness has virtually been decriminalized (Fig. 3.10), but has also been marked in England and Wales. Discussions with police and other officials indicate that these apparent falls may reflect changes in policy rather than a real improvement in the situation. The latter is judged by some to have to have deteriorated substantially. However the well-regarded British Crime Survey supports the view that public perceptions about rising crime may be either exaggerated or simply wrong. An analysis of study findings for alcohol-related disorder in England and Wales has indicated that this declined between 1995 and 1999:

> 'The overall rate fell significantly (by 21%) between 1995 and 1997, remaining stable between 1997 and 1999. This pattern is consistent with the overall trend in violence over that period.' (Budd 2003, p.iv).

Fresh evidence emerged in October 2005 showing that there had been a 6% rise in alcohol-related violent crime in the year ending in June of that year.

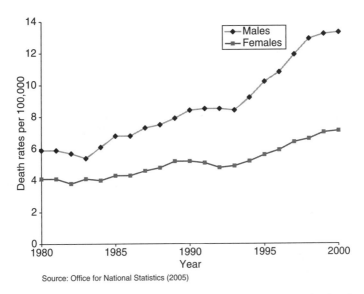

Source: Office for National Statistics (2005)

Fig. 3.7 Death rates (per 100, 000) from alcohol-related diseases in England and Wales (1980–2000)

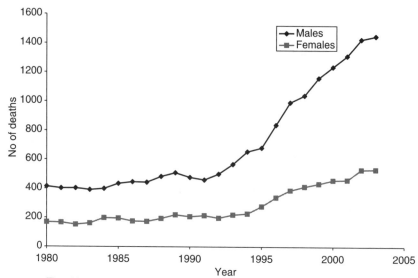

The table may underestimate the number of alcohol-related deaths as conditions such as alcohol attributable cancers are excluded from these analyses.

Source: Alcohol Information Scotland (2005)

Fig. 3.8 Number of alcohol-related deaths in Scotland (1980–2003)

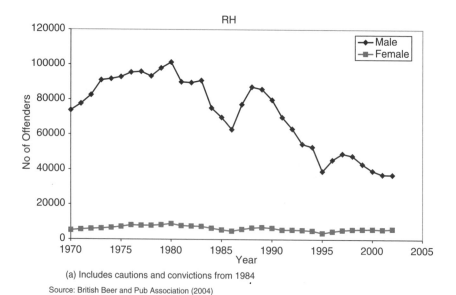

(a) Includes cautions and convictions from 1984

Source: British Beer and Pub Association (2004)

Fig. 3.9 Drunkenness offenders in England and Wales (1970–2002)

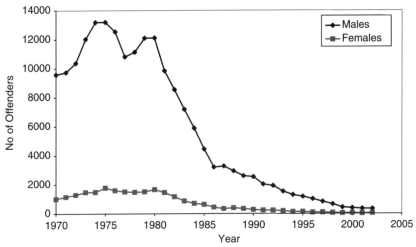

(a) From 1970 to 1978—numbers found guilty or convicted of drunkenness; thereafter persons with a main charge proved for drunkenness.
(b) From 1988 the total includes a number of cases where the sex of the offender was not documented.
Source: British Beer and Pub Association (2004)

Fig. 3.10 Drunkenness offenders in Scotland (1970–2002)

This was in contrast with an overall fall in crime. The British Crime Survey suggested that crime had fallen over the same period (Travis 2005a).

Budd (2003) reports that those most at risk of experiencing alcohol-related violence (as victims) were males aged 16–29 years, single people, the unemployed, frequent pub and night club patrons and heavy drinkers. Budd also notes that 19% of all reported incidents of alcohol-related violence (and 34% of violence at the hands of strangers) occurred in or around a pub, bar, or club. Additional research for the Home Office (2003) showed that binge drinkers were more likely than other young adults to commit crimes. Thirty nine per cent of the binge drinkers aged 18–24 years studied had committed an offence in the past year. It was also concluded that connection between drinking and crime was particularly strong for violent crime:

'Qualitative research found that most of the young adults had experienced assaults fighting while out drinking. They identified an array of factors they felt contributed to the link between alcohol and crime and disorder. There were four broad groups: effects of binge drinking, attitudes and motivation, social and peer norms, and the drinking environment.' (p. 1)

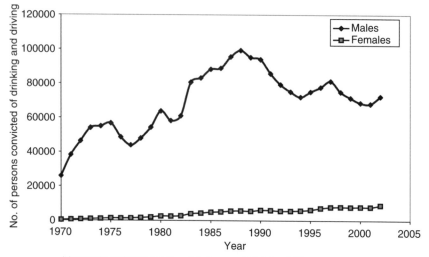

(a) 1967 Road Safety Act came into force on 9 October 1968.
(b) 1981 Transport Act introduced, evidential breath testing from 6 May 1983.

The figures cover people for whom drinking and driving was the principal offence
dealt with at a court appearance. They are lower (by between 14 and 20%) than
the total number of drinking and driving offences because several offences may
be dealt with at one court appearance when drinking and driving is not
necessarily the principal offence.

Source: British Beer and Pub Association (2004)

Fig. 3.11 Persons convicted of drinking and driving in England and Wales (1970–2002)

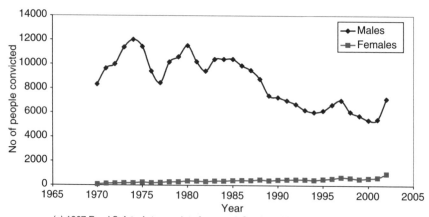

(a) 1967 Road Safety Act came into force on 9 October 1968.
(b) 1981 Transport Act introduced, evidential breath testing from 6 May 1983.

The figures cover people for whom drinking and driving was the principal offence dealt
with at a court appearance. They are lower (by between 14 and 20%) than the total
number of drinking and driving offences because several offences may be dealt with
at one court appearance when drinking and driving is not necessarily the principal
offence.

Source: British Beer and Pub Association (2004)

Fig. 3.12 Persons convicted of drinking and driving in Scotland (1970–2002)

One area where there is general agreement that there has been improvement is that of alcohol-impaired or drunk driving. This has decreased substantially since 1990 in England and Wales (Fig. 3.11) and since the 1970s in Scotland (Fig. 3.12). It should, however, be noted from these figures that there has recently been an increase in this form of offence throughout Britain.

Chapter 4

Alcohol policy in the United Kingdom

As noted in previous chapters, it has been evident that alcohol has had distinctive and problematic characteristics for a very long time. On the one hand, it is accepted as the major legal recreational drug of much of the world. On the other hand, its consumption has widespread adverse effects. The response of governments since the sixteenth century has been to attempt to balance the popularity and positive effects of alcohol with its associated problems. The continual rise and fall of alcohol consumption has been accompanied by alternating periods of relaxation and restriction of the availability and price of drink.

Current policies on alcohol have been set out by policy documents covering Scotland, Northern Ireland, and England and to some degree, Wales. Each of these documents expresses the wish that the problems associated with heavy drinking should be reduced by consistent and coherent action on the part of government departments.

The UK's 'classified' alcohol policy

During 1982 a number of researchers, medical authorities, and others received unexpected postal deliveries. These contained copies of an orange-covered report that had been printed in Sweden by the late Kettil Bruun, a well known and widely respected Finnish researcher. This document was a leaked report on alcohol policy that had been produced by a UK Government 'think tank' known as the Central Policy Review Staff (1979). The report had concluded that the best way to curb the UK's levels of alcohol problems was to use tax to increase the price of alcoholic beverages. The report, which outlined the massive economic costs of alcohol problems, was considered to be so politically 'hot' that the newly elected Prime Minister Margaret Thatcher had it covered by the Official Secrets Act. Since this curious development, alcohol policies have been discussed by several agencies and a considerable body of evidence on the impact of alternative policies has been produced. This is considered further in Chapter 7.

Wales

An overall strategy for drug and alcohol misuse in Wales was published in 1996. This was primarily designed to address both prevention of the misuse of alcohol and illicit drugs and to provide treatment, support, and rehabilitation for those in need of such assistance (Welsh Office 1996). The joint consideration of alcohol and other drugs in Wales has been consolidated by the Welsh Assembly. This approach has been set out with the following four aims. (The National Assembly for Wales 2000):

'Children, young people, and adults
To help children, young people, and adults resist substance misuse in order to achieve their full potential in society, and to promote sensible drinking in the context of a healthy lifestyle.
Families and communities
To protect families and communities from anti-social behaviour and health risks related to substance misuse.
Treatment
To enable people with substance misuse problems to overcome them and live healthy and fulfilling lives and in the case of offenders, crime-free lives.
Availability
To stifle the availability of illegal drugs on our streets and inappropriate availability of other substances.'

A number of those working in the health and social services have expressed the view to the authors that in practice, Welsh policy has been far more focussed on illegal drugs than upon alcohol. In addition, it should be noted that in some areas, notably liquor licensing, policy in Wales in still dictated by Westminster.

Northern Ireland

A wide-ranging *Strategy for Reducing Alcohol-Related Harm* for Northern Ireland was published in 2000. This was designed to reduce 'all types of alcohol-related harm'. The strategy gave prominence to health promotion and a range of fairly mild harm minimisation measures. The strategy aimed to encourage sensible drinking, to provide and improve treatment services, protect the community (from alcohol-related anti-social and criminal behaviour), develop information and research, and to implement and manage the chosen policies. It emphasised partnership and openness to innovative approaches. It undertook to:

'Work with the drinks industry to address areas of common concern. These include the development of agreed policies for product marketing and policies for distribution which promote safer drinking environments.' (Department of Health, Social Services and Public Safety 2000 p.15).

The strategy also embraced the policy of reducing access to alcohol by under-age drinkers. In November 2005 the Government announced plans for liberalizing opening hours in Northern Ireland from 2007. These did not include a proposal that 24 hour drinking would be introduced. Nevertheless it did propose to extend permitted bar opening hours to: '2 a.m. from Monday to Saturday, with no change to the existing midnight closing time on Sundays'. (McCambridge 2005). These plans were to be subject to a three month consultation period.

Scotland

In Scotland a white paper identified a number of objectives in dealing with the problems of alcohol in 1999. *Plan for Action on Alcohol Problems* was published three years later (Scottish Executive 2002). This committed the Scottish Executive to reducing the level of alcohol-related problems throughout Scotland. The plan has a number of clear targets. As noted by Crombie *et al.* (2005), these include reducing the numbers of men and women drinking more than 'sensible drinking levels' from: '33% to 31% for men between 1995 and 2005 and to 29% by 2010; 13% to 12% for women between 1995 and 2005 and to 11% by 2010'. In addition it was also planned to reduce alcohol consumption among 12–15-year-olds. The plan identified a number of key indicators by which the impact of policy should be assessed. These include binge drinking, drinking patterns, and alcohol-related mortality. Sadly at the time of writing there appears to be little sign that these objectives are being met.

The Licensing (Scotland) Bill was published on March 1st, 2005. This was launched with the claim that it would sever the link between binge drinking and crime. This legislation sets out to (i) Reform outdated licensing laws; (ii) Tackle under-age drinking; (iii) Crack down on binge drinking; (iv) Involve communities. Mr Tavish Scott, Scotland's Minister for Finance and Public service Reform said:

'Our current licensing system dates back to the 1970s—it does not reflect Scottish society in the 21st century. That is why the Executive is bringing forward legislation to reform our outdated licensing laws...We want a robust licensing system which will improve health and break the link between excessive drinking and crime. There is no doubt our record here makes grim reading...Nearly three-quarters of the assailants in violent crimes were reported to be under the influence of drink... One third of prisoners said they would not be in prison if they had not been drinking... Young people—aged between 16 and 24—in Scotland drink more than any other age group... 59 per cent of 15 year olds drink alcopops and 24 per cent claim to have bought alcohol from a shop; and . . . The annual cost of alcohol misuse on the NHS in Scotland was £110.5 million and the total cost to Scottish society is estimated to be £1.1 billion.

Those shocking statistics illustrate exactly why doing nothing is simply not an option—alcohol-fuelled violence and anti-social behaviour is a real and visible problem across Scotland and must be tackled. That is why we are taking immediate and sustained action for the long-term.'

Mr Scott said the Licensing Bill would reform outdated licensing laws by:

Establishing a clear, effective and mandatory national framework which will include standard national licence conditions covering key issues; abolishing the outdated system of seven licences and statutory opening hours, replacing them with two new licences—personal and premises licence; a sensible 'premises by premises' approach to opening hours authorised by local Licensing Boards in line with the new licensing principles coupled with a statutory presumption against 24 hour opening; and emphasis on mandatory training and tougher enforcement—wider range of sanctions and new Licensing Standards Officers (LSOs).

He said it would tackle under-age drinking by: 'a requirement for all licensees to operate on a no-proof no-sale basis; a requirement for on-sales premises who want to allow access by children to set out their plans in their operating plan for approval by the Board—emphasis on making family access easy to suitable premises: overhaul of under-age drinking offences.

It would tackle binge drinking by: a crackdown on 'irresponsible promotional activities'—a new policy which will ensure drinks have to be sold at the same price for at least 48 hours and a ban on specific irresponsible promotions that encourage binge and speed drinking like two-for-ones. And the legislation would protect communities by: a new approach to overprovision for all licensed premises—boards to conduct overprovision assessments and block licences in saturated hot-spots; any person can object or make representations to a licence application—no unnecessary definitions of 'neighbour'; key role of mediation for LSOs between trade and community to help sort out problems at local level; local forums with community representation with role of commenting on Board's proposed policies.'

To protect the unique nature of clubs and their place in communities, the Scottish Ministers would be provided with a regulatory power to exempt very small clubs should they meet certain conditions set out in the Bill. In general this would mean that these clubs would be exempt from the requirement to have a premises manager, and exemption from the 'overprovision assessment' that would be carried out by local authority Licensing Boards. Mr Scott added:

'This devolved government recognises that most people in Scotland can and do drink sensibly—and we want to help promote this kind of approach to alcohol. I have no doubts responsible drinking can be part of a healthy, happy and sociable lifestyle . . . .

But I am sure most people will agree Scotland has an appalling record on alcohol—the health and social problems irresponsible and excessive drinking can cause are well-known to all of us. Doing nothing is not an option if we are to address that...

We are determined to put in place a licensing system that contributes to a safer, stronger Scotland. It will also ensure that 21st Century Scotland has reformed licensing laws, laws which can respond to changing habits and behaviour and support the drinks industry from producer to consumer...

There is no doubt irresponsible drinks promotions fuel the violence and anti-social behaviour which blight communities in Scotland. It is a simple fact that some promotions encourage many people to drink more alcohol—and they therefore help contribute to our grim record in this area...

By removing promotions like these we move closer to protecting young people and making our town and city centres safer—helping to make Scotland a safer place to visit, live in and socialise...

There are too many licensed premises in some areas—which can be the root of problems being experienced by many communities where there has been no coherent overall policy in place. We will make it easier for a wider range of people from local communities to have a say in the grant of licences...

We will overhaul the regulations on under-age drinking to ensure the system offers the maximum level of protection possible to children and young people. There will be a no-proof, no-sale approach everywhere...

Crucially, we will also establish a clear and effective mandatory national framework which will include standard conditions...

All of this adds up to the most comprehensive and ambitious package of licensing reform Scotland has ever seen. It will take our licensing laws into the 21st Century—and provide a platform to tackle many of the problems alcohol can cause in our society.'

Health Minister Andy Kerr said:

'Harmful drinking is currently taking an unacceptable toll on Scottish society and firm action is required to change drinking cultures...

Excessive drinking carries with it serious health and other consequences and I am particularly concerned about the increase in binge drinking which is harmful both to the individual concerned and to society more generally...

These legislative proposals will contribute to the range of work we're doing to reduce harmful drinking. Attitudes won't change overnight, but the proposed measures, particularly those aimed at underage drinking and binge drinking generally, will make an enormous contribution to tackling the problem.' (Scottish Executive 2005).

At the time of writing the Scottish plan was being revised, subject to a consultation process.

England

The Government did not act so rapidly in producing an alcohol policy for England. The Prime Minister's Cabinet Office, having consulted widely with a variety of people concerned with alcohol issues, produced an *Interim Analytic Report*. This consisted of a review of evidence on alcohol matters in the summer of 2003 (Cabinet Office Prime Minister's Strategy Unit 2003). The review gave a concise overview of evidence related to the extent of alcohol problems in Britain as well as some comment on the impact of alternative alcohol control policies, such as alcohol education and taxation. This review was generally well-received, even though, predictably, it did not satisfy everybody. The final version of the Cabinet Office's report was published in March 2004 as the *Alcohol Harm Reduction Strategy for England* (sometimes known by the unfortunate acronym "AHRSE") (Cabinet Office Prime Minister's Strategy Unit 2004).

This strategy sets out the following elements:

'Better education and communication

The strategy includes measures aimed at achieving a long term change in attitudes to irresponsible drinking and behaviour, including: making the sensible drinking message easier to understand and apply; targeting messages at those most at risk, including binge- and chronic drinkers; providing better information for consumers, both on products and at the point of sale; providing alcohol education in schools that can change attitudes and behaviour; providing more support and advice for employers; and reviewing the code of practice for TV advertising to ensure that it does not target young drinkers or glamorise irresponsible behaviour.

Improving health and treatment services

The strategy proposes a number of measures to improve early identification and treatment of alcohol problems. These measures include: improved training of staff to increase awareness of likely signs of alcohol misuse; piloting schemes to find out whether earlier identification and treatment of those with alcohol problems can improve health and lead to longer-term savings; carrying out a national audit of the demand for and provision of alcohol treatment services, to identify any gaps between demand and provision; and better help for the most vulnerable such as homeless people, drug addicts, the mentally ill and young people. They often have multiple problems and need clear pathways for treatment from a variety of sources.

Combating alcohol-related crime and disorder

The strategy proposes a series of measures to address the problems of those town and city centres that are blighted by alcohol misuse at weekends. These include: greater use of exclusion orders to ban those causing trouble from pubs and clubs or entire town centres; greater use of the newly fixed penalty fines for anti-social behaviour; working with licensees to ensure better enforcement of existing rules on under-age drinking and serving people who are already drunk. We will also work in partnership with the industry to reduce anti-social behaviours—issues to be addressed may include layout of pubs and availability of seating, managing crime and disorder in city centres and improved information on safe drinking in pubs; and in addition to local initiatives, the Security Industry Authority (SIA) will begin the licensing of door supervisors with effect from March 2004.

Working with the alcohol industry

The strategy will build on the good practice of some existing initiatives (such as the Manchester City Centre Safe Scheme) and involve the alcohol industry in new initiatives at both national level (drinks producers) and local level (restaurants, pubs and clubs).

At a national level, a social responsibility charter for drinks producers, will strongly encourage drinks companies to: pledge not to manufacture products irresponsibly—for example, no products that appeal to under-age drinkers or that encourage people to drink well over recommended limits; ensure that advertising does not promote or condone irresponsible or excessive drinking; put the sensible drinking message clearly on the bottle alongside information about unit content; move to packaging products in safer materials—for example, alternatives to glass bottles; and make a financial contribution to a fund that pays for new schemes to address alcohol misuse at national and local levels, such as providing information and alternative facilities for young people.'

The *Alcohol Harm Reduction Strategy for England* is a strange document, differing in a number of striking ways from the previous year's Interim Analytic Report by the Cabinet Office. The Strategy was not nearly as well received as the previous year's Cabinet Office document. It has been widely criticised by medical authorities and social scientists (e.g. Drummond 2004, M.A. Plant 2004, Room 2004a, Hall 2005a,b, Luty 2005). Remarkably the Alcohol Harm Reduction Strategy for England has neither specific targets nor much money to back it. It does provide some useful evidence about the scale of alcohol problems, but is deficient in a number of areas. A number of topics that were included in the *Interim Analytic Report* had simply vanished or were edited into insignificance. These include alcohol and family violence, the ineffectiveness of alcohol education and the value of taxation as a control policy. Furthermore leaked Whitehall documents indicate that evidence of a link between alcohol and 19,000 sexual assaults per year was also expunged (Leppard and Winnett 2005). The section dealing with alcohol treatment is written as if most of the extensive available international evidence on this subject did not exist. A psychiatrist with long experience of working in the alcohol field commented to the authors 'It looks as if the industry has edited this, knocking out anything that threatens them or would reduce alcohol consumption.' This comment and many of the other criticisms of the strategy document were prompted by the fact that in spite of having reviewed a considerable amount of evidence, the Cabinet Office Team finally produced an *Alcohol Harm Reduction Strategy for England* that highlights control policies acknowledged by most credible scientists as being useless or of very little value. These are alcohol education and voluntary agreements with the beverage alcohol industry. The strategy document is also remarkable for the seventeen times it mentions the alcohol industry's organisation, the Portman Group.

The Prime Minister's foreword to the strategy acknowledges that alcohol problems cost roughly £20 billion per year in England. It endorses harm minimisation through 'partnership between government, local authorities, police, industry, and the public themselves'.

The Strategy identifies its main elements as being the provision of better education and communication, improving health and treatment services, and combating alcohol-related disorder through exclusion orders to ban trouble makers from pubs, fixed penalty fines for anti-social behaviour, better enforcement of rules on under-age drinking, and serving drunks. The Strategy also states that:

> 'issues to be addressed may include layout of pubs and availability of seating, managing crime and disorder in city centres and improved information on safe drinking in pubs.'

The Strategy also promised the production of a social responsibility charter that would encourage the beverage alcohol industry to be socially responsible, adopt safer packaging materials, and contribute to a fund to pay for new schemes 'to address alcohol misuse at national and local levels such as providing information and alternative facilities for young people'. It noted that participation in schemes of this type was voluntary.

The clear view of most British (and some overseas) social scientists and medical authorities was and remains that the Strategy does not set out a credible means of significantly reducing either heavy drinking or the problems associated with this type of behaviour. Indeed, one eminent researcher has quipped that the Strategy emphasises exactly those policies that any serious authority would toss into the garbage heap. Luty (2005) has commented:

'One of the most ludicrous lines in the harm reduction strategy states: 'there is no direct correlation between drinking and the harm experienced or caused by individuals'. An equally bizarre statement in the strategy states: 'evidence (which) suggested that using price as a key lever risked major unintended side effects', presumably to Mr Blair's re-election hopes.' (p.401).

Another statement in the strategy could embarrass drinks manufactures if interpreted literally. This is the request for them to pledge 'not to manufacture products ... that appeal to under-age drinkers'. The latter appear to like beer, wine, and spirits!

The Academy of Medical Sciences (2004b) reacted to the publication of the *Alcohol Harm Reduction Strategy* with a press release that stated:

'The evidence presented in the recent Academy report, *Calling Time*, shows that even a modest 10 per cent increase in the price of alcoholic beverages could reduce deaths from alcohol-related conditions by up to 37 per cent and would be highly effective at dealing with under-age drinking ... Measures such as reducing the availability of alcohol, reducing EU travel allowances and reducing the statutory blood alcohol concentration for drivers must also be considered.'

The formulation of recent alcohol policies within the UK has been predicated by a governmental wish to cooperate and agree with the beverage alcohol industry. The latter wields enormous economic and political power and appears to have dominated much of the policy-making process. In Ireland the Strategic Task Force on Alcohol broke ranks with the industry when it identified reducing the general level of alcohol consumption by taxation and the introduction of random breath testing as key policies. The drinks industry disagreed with these policy choices and produced a minority report of their own.

The current chosen alcohol policies of the constituent parts of the United Kingdom can be described as 'harm minimisation lite'. They appear to be the products of processes or reasoning that give pre-eminence to consensus rather than to effectiveness. The implications of this and some of the evidence about what might really work are considered in the final chapter of this book.

It would be logical to devise a national policy on alcohol or any health issue that is consistent and based upon the best scientific evidence. The next chapter sets out some of the strange events surrounding discussion of Government plans to liberalise liquor licensing arrangements at a time when alcohol-related problems are rising and scientific, medical, and public concern about these problems is growing. The current Government intention of expanding bar opening hours in England and Wales is in remarkable contrast to the Licensing Act of 1872, the Metropolitan Police Act of 1893, and the Defence of the Realm Act of 1914. These acts had restricted bar opening hours in order to reduce drunkenness and public disorder.

As noted earlier, it has been suggested that alcohol consumption and its associated problems rise and fall in long waves. British history suggests that nothing really inspires the introduction of effective alcohol control policies better than a crisis. This has been demonstrated by the Gin Craze, the upsurge of alcohol problems in the later nineteenth century and concern about drunkenness impeding the country's military capabilities during the First World War. Not even the most powerful vested interests were able to resist the pressure for reform. Controls were even acknowledged as being in the national interest by some of those associated with the drinks industry, such as Sir Edgar Sanders. He put patriotism before the profits of his industry. This sadly contrasts with the approach of some of his successors.

Chapter 5

Bar wars: media frenzy and licensing chaos

'The late hour at which they remain open at night is a very great source of evil. Many persons are tempted to go there and led on, step by step, to criminal or immoral proceedings, which they would not be led into if there were no place for them to remain away from their homes at night.' (Sir Richard Mayne, Chief Commissioner of the Metropolitan Police (1853) cited by Kneale 1999 p.340)

This chapter records some of the events and media reports that have related to the recent debate about the extension of liquor licensing in England and Wales. This makes very uncomfortable reading for anybody who believes that the UK's alcohol policy should be mainly designed to protect public health and safety. It would appear that other considerations have been at work. Proposals to liberalize liquor licensing arrangements in England and Wales were set out in a White Paper (a formal discussion document) 'Time for reform: proposals for the modernisation of our licensing laws', in April 2000. The Licensing Bill was introduced in Parliament on November 14th, 2002. On July 10th, 2003 this received the Royal assent, becoming the Licensing Act 2003 in spite of Liberal Democrat opposition. A key component of the new legislation was the introduction of the following:

'Flexible opening hours for premises with the potential for up to 24-hour opening, seven days a week, subject to consideration of the impact on local residents, businesses and the expert opinion of a range of authorities in relation to the licensing objectives. This will help to minimise public disorder resulting from fixed closing times.' (Department of Culture, Media and Sport 2005).

The Tourism Division of the DCMS took over responsibility for liquor licensing from the Home office in 2001. This change was controversial:

'It certainly led to heated exchanges between the Home Office, troubled by the possible repercussions of flexible hours for crime and disorder and the DCMS.' (Light 2005c)

The Right Honourable Tessa Jowell, MP, the Culture Secretary, addressed the 10th Anniversary Conference of the Association of Licensed and Multiple Retailers in 2002. She stated:

'Pubs are at the heart of our communities, both in town and country. They bring a great deal of enjoyment and social contact for people of all ages...But our licensing laws speak for another decade, not our own. I am determined that we deliver on our promises and bring forward our new legislation to modernise our licensing laws as soon as possible.'

She went on to state that the new arrangements (including flexible hours, with the potential for up to 24-hour opening) would eliminate problems of disorder and disturbance associated with fixed and artificially early closing times (Department of Culture, Media and Sport 2002). This weighty assertion was not justified with reference to any evidence, nor was it supported by a single credible scientist. This statement was surprising given Tessa Jowell's previous involvement with alcohol issues. At an earlier stage in her distinguished career she had been a social worker in an alcohol treatment clinic in London. In fact, the belief that 'flexible' bar closing hours would reduce either heavy drinking or disorder is open to dispute. A number of commentators have suggested that this would simply foster 'circuit drinking' as bar patrons might successively move from earlier closing venues to those remaining open later.

As outlined in the previous chapter, Britain's alcohol policies have recently been subject to severe criticism. The *Alcohol Harm Reduction Strategy for England* was published in 2004. This document omitted much that was included in a far better earlier review of evidence. The latter had, in the views of many commentators, been 'sexed down'. Sections on the value of taxation and licensing controls and the general ineffectiveness of alcohol education was amongst that having been edited out (Cabinet Office Prime Minister's Strategy Unit 2003, 2004). (See comments by Drummond 2004, M. A. Plant 2004, Room 2004a, Winnett and Leppard 2005).

It should be noted that there are no plans to introduce 24-hour licensing in Scotland or in Northern Ireland. Even so, it has been reported that some 24-hour licences may be granted 'in exceptional circumstances' in Scotland after new laws take effect in 2007 (Macdonell 2005). New, more flexible, Scottish licensing arrangements were recommended by the Nicholson Committee (2003). Even so, Cathy Jamieson, Scotland's Justice Minister, a Labour MSP, has stated that there was 'neither the desire nor the evidence to support' this (BBC News Online 2003). Sheriff Nicholson has expressed the view that changing Scottish liquor licensing laws will not change drinking culture. This view runs counter to that voiced by Tessa Jowell and other Government ministers in relation to licensing in England and Wales. Debate in the Scottish Parliament on the subject of liquor licensing has not been without controversy. An editorial in the *Scotsman* described this as 'shambolic, confused, reactive and lacking in strategic direction'. (Scotsman 2005a). There have been several prominent players in the recent national debate about liquor licensing. The public tone of this has been set by the mass media. Because of this the next section provides a select sample of the media coverage of this controversial topic before reporting some of the statements and actions of other players.

The media response

By the end of 2004 public attention and media interest were becoming increasingly concerned about the social disorder, violence, and other problems associated with heavy drinking and intoxication, especially in town and city centres during weekend evenings. The prospect of liberalised licensing arrangements increasingly came under fire from all quarters and a sustained and quite remarkable onslaught against these changes continued throughout 2005. Some of the main events during this period, largely through reports in newspapers, are described in this chapter. A feature of media coverage has been the fact that newspapers with widely varied political orientations joined forces to support a common cause. Such agreement is very rare in relation to any topic. Moreover, the press has mounted a vigorous and outspoken campaign against Government plans. The *Daily Mail* in particular, ran a concerted campaign opposing the liberalization. Media interest built upon and probably amplified a moral panic about binge drinking that had been running for several months.

The media response has been aggressive and wide-ranging. *The Mail on Sunday* bore the following front page headline in 2005: 'Exposed: Mandarin Ally of Alcohol Bosses'. The article that followed stated that Mr Andrew Cunningham, a senior civil servant (or 'mandarin'), at the Department of Culture, Media and Sport (DCMS) had called critics of the extended licensing arrangements 'extremists'. Mr Cunningham, it was noted, is in charge of the new licensing policy within his department. He had allegedly been the subject of a complaint for calling opponents of more liberal licensing 'nanny staters'. The latter is a term usually associated with right-wing British politicians who oppose state intervention on social or health issues. *The Mail on Sunday* also reported that:

> 'Mr Cunningham attended many pub and alcohol parties and alcohol trade conferences cocktail parties and lavish dinners thrown by the drinks industry which has spent a fortune on a lobbying campaign to win support for 24-hour drinking.'

This edition of the paper also cited several Labour politicians, including Mr Frank Dobson (former Secretary of State for Health) criticising the proposed licensing changes and the role of the DCMS (Walters and Lewis 2005). On the same day the *Sunday Times* printed a front page story revealing that leaked documents showed that the former Home Secretary Mr David Blunkett and his senior officials had attempted to block the Government's plans to liberalize licensing arrangements. (Blunkett had reportedly called the planned changes 'a leap in the dark'). These objections were reportedly blocked by Tessa Jowell and the DCMS (Winnett and Leppard 2005). The authors also noted that: 'A consultation document by Blair's Strategy Unit was redrafted to remove evidence of a link between drink and 19,000 sex assaults a year and the adverse effect a 24-hour opening might have on local residents'. This is a reference to the widely criticised *Alcohol Harm Reduction Strategy for England* (Winnett and Leppard 2005). It was also claimed by Winnet and Leppard that: '(Tessa) Jowell wanted to change the definition of binge drinking to downplay the extent of the problem'. This article provided details of serious disagreements between the DCMS (strongly in favour of licensing liberalization and the Home Office (strongly opposed to such innovations). Mr David Davis, the Conservative Party's Shadow Home Secretary stated:

'This leak shows the Government's own fears that 24-hour drinking will actually increase violent crime. The new law should be delayed until these problems have been brought under control.' (Winnett and Leppard 2005 p.2).

The *Daily Mail* printed a front page headline: 'Boozing Britain: another cover-up'. This newspaper reported that the Prime Minister's office has suppressed a:

'second damning report on the binge drinking culture. Tony Blair had been warned that a million drunks a year already besiege casualty departments even before the introduction of 24-hour drinking.'

The same edition of the paper reported that local councils in England are 'threatening Tessa Jowell with a High Court challenge over the extra costs of overseeing the new rules for pubs and clubs'. (Daily Mail 2005a) This edition also published two colour maps. These showed that the concentration of licensed premises in central London coincided with the geographical distribution of violent crime. A separate article in the same edition stated that the liberalisation of Scottish licensing had been a disaster and that Government policy in relation to English licensing was 'creating a climate of unfettered irresponsibility' (Dickson-Wright 2005). The *Guardian* reported that:

'Ministers responsible for new licensing laws were under pressure to delay plans for 24-hour drinking yesterday amid new calculations showing that the measures could cost councils an extra £40 million a year.'

The Association of Chief Police Officers (ACPO) was also cited as believing that the new arrangements would increase anti-social behaviour. In addition this report quoted the disapproval by one of the authors of the appointment by the DCMS of an employee of the Portman Group to the Alcohol Education & Research Council (see Room 2004b) (Hetherington 2005).

There was another media flare up in August 2005, following the closing date for the submission of applications for new liquor licences. This renewal of interest was prompted by the publication of concerns by ACPO and senior Judges. These are detailed later in this chapter. This renewal of vocal hostility to the extension of bar hours prompted *The Times* newspaper to run the front page headline: 'Late drinking law in danger as rebellion gathers pace'. *The Mail on Sunday* published a report on August 14th 2005 alleging that:

> 'Key Labour figures who drew up the new 24-hour drinking laws received thousands of pounds in foreign junkets and hospitality from the alcohol industry.'

This report related to the alleged activities of the All-Party Beer Group or 'Beer Club'. The latter had reportedly received funding from beverage alcohol companies. Mark Field, a Conservative MP who was a member of this committee has reportedly claimed:

> 'We did our best to ensure the concerns of residential populations nearby *(pubs)* were properly addressed. The issues of binge drinking and anti-social behaviour were raised...But the Labour side was packed with people who stayed silent throughout the proceedings or stood up for the interests of the large-scale alcohol and entertainment industry. The pub and bar giants are driving out smaller, family-run, independent outlets by appealing to the lowest common denominator.'

The Mail on Sunday continued its campaign with another long article. This reported the following:

> 'The political storm over 24-hour drinking intensified last night as it was revealed that the 'independent' researchers behind Labour's controversial plans have been in the pay of brewing bosses.'

This report alleged that researchers Dr Peter Marsh and Ms Kate Fox had been influential in 'arguing that longer pub hours would lead to less binge drinking and street violence.' (Oliver 2005a). This belief has little support among academic alcohol researchers. Marsh and Fox do not appear to have published any work on the subject of pubs or alcohol-related violence in scientific journals.

Polly Toynbee (2005), writing in the *Guardian* in August declared that the only way to curb Britain's alcohol problems was to put the price up. Magnus Linklater (2005) in *The Times* wrote scathingly as follows:

> 'It is not just the idiocy of it all, it is the serial incompetence. We watch, aghast, as yet another government measure unravels before our eyes, its intentions confused, its

execution bungled, its operation opposed by the very people who will be required to implement it. In the face of flaws that loom ever larger as the deadline approaches, ministers retreat behind political mantras that sound more feeble each time they are repeated.

It is hard to find a reputable voice prepared to speak up for the plans to extend licensing hours in England and Wales. Police chiefs, judges, local authorities, a growing proportion of the voting public, and even some leading publicans have voiced their objections in the face of a binge-drinking culture that has become a national blight. Yesterday, another plank in the tottering structure of the Government's defence fell away when *The Times* revealed a huge rise in the number of pubs, clubs, and restaurants planning to extend their opening hours, after a rush in applications before the August 6th deadline. Far from a small minority seeking to take advantage of the new regime, up to two-thirds of all licensed premises and 90 per cent of bars are planning to cater for drinking up to midnight during the week and 2 a.m. at weekends. That adds up to around 130,000, most of them in the very city centres that have become no-go areas at night for the non-fighting, non-vomiting, non-urinating public. Ministers assured us that the number of pubs applying for late-night licences would be small, and would reduce the pressure at closing time. The figures fly in the face of that claim. Instead of an 11 p.m. surge, we are a heading for an alcohol-fuelled midnight surge instead.

With only two weeks to go for objections to be recorded by September 4, the number so far received is low—some 20,000 for the whole of the country. There will be more, of course, but the last-minute flood has meant that it has been difficult for residents to hear about, let alone object to, an extension of hours. Yet this is the only means that local councils have for opposing an application, given the intent of the legislation is to encourage, rather than constrain, longer drinking hours. If there is no formal objection, then a licence must be approved. A councillor or local environmental body can lodge an objection, but many of them were away on holiday when the August deadline loomed. Police have the right to object, but they have to gather evidence showing the adverse effects of giving a particular drinking establishment longer opening hours and have only limited time to do so.

Finally, there has to be a 28-day period for objections to be heard after an application has been made. People claiming that they have been denied that can take their case to local magistrates, thus removing the decision from the very councils that are meant to be making them. This sounds absurd.' (p.19).

The Mail on Sunday, continuing to campaign vigorously against the new licensing regulations, printed a sensational front page headline on August 28th 2005: 'Now it's 24-hour drinking for Kids'. This stated that:

'Thousands of children will be allowed into rowdy late-night drinking establishments thanks to Labour's controversial licensing laws... Alcohol industry lawyers are exploiting small print in the legislation to remove current restrictions that keep youngsters under 14 out of pubs, clubs and bars. (Oliver 2005b).

The Mail on Sunday reported on August 4th, 2005 that the new laws to extend bar opening hours were drawn up during a series of meetings, some of which took place in the offices of the British Beer and Pub Association in 2002 and 2003:

> The (licensing) advisory group is chaired by Andrew Cunningham, the Culture Department civil servant in charge of licensing. Mr Cunningham has faced accusations of being too close to the drinks industry... One representative who asked not to be named, said: 'I was one of the few people opposed to the drinking free-for-all. I thought it odd that we were meeting at what was effect-ively the HQ of Britain's pub trade'.... Conservative MP Mark Field, whose City of Westminster seat includes the West End bar district, said: 'These meetings reinforce the impression that the whole process was driven by the industry. We are talking about well financed groups which stand to gain or lose millions of pounds from this legislation.' (Oliver 2005c).

Press criticism of Governmental insistence that it was pressing ahead with the licensing liberalisation was re-emphasised by the following scathing leader comment in the *Guardian* on September 22nd, 2005:

> The 2003 Licensing Act has been nothing but trouble for the Labour government. Public opinion never wanted the act in the first place. Now that the liberalisation of drinking law is on the statute book, public opinion likes it even less. In a poll this month, nearly two-thirds of voters said they oppose the plans. Only the under-25s, whose drinking is the source of much of the wider anxiety, want bars and pubs open longer. Police, doctors and judges all think the change is a change for the worse. Yet still the government ploughs on, as stubbornly determined to prove the people wrong about the drinking culture of the inner cities as about the invasion of Iraq. Are they mad?
>
> To listen to culture secretary Tessa Jowell this week, it is hard not to think so. More than 30,000 objections have been lodged to applications for extended drinking hours by more than 60,000 bars when the new law finally comes into force on November 24. As proof of popular distaste for a law goes, this is surely about as massive as it gets. Yet, in an interview this week, Ms Jowell claimed that this wave of popular outrage was proof, not of the misjudgment of the law, but of its success. That so many of the public were using their right to object to longer opening hours was, she said, 'people power' in action. It was a comment worthy of Marie Antoinette.
>
> Now, nevertheless, Whitehall appears to have made a concession to the public mood. Until now, the government has said that the act would remain in force for a year before a review of its effects was carried out. This week, ministers announced that the review will begin next February, just three months after the new system comes into effect.
>
> In so far as this change implies the government is listening to the hostile clamour about the new law, this decision is welcome. But it is really an admission of failure. It is an attempt to give an impression of responsiveness while not addressing the

seriousness of the excessive drinking problem. A far better approach is to delay the general implementation and to give the liberalisation of the licensing laws, a well-intentioned and desirable reform in some ways, a trial run in a number of local authority areas. That way the practical lessons can be learned without inflicting a flawed system (if that is what it is) on the police, courts, hospitals and citizens of the country as a whole. Ms Jowell should swallow her pride. Ministers should brace themselves to take a real decision on the licensing laws, not a phoney one. They might find they have never been so popular.' (Guardian 2005a)

A development occurred in late October 2005 that was very embarrassing for the Government. This was described in a report published in the *Observer*:

'The drinks industry is planning a ruthless campaign of economic incentives and psychological tricks to get customers to drink as much as possible when licensing laws are relaxed, the *Observer* can reveal.

Managers of massive 'vertical drinking' pubs are being offered bonuses worth up to £20,000 a year if they beat targets as the industry moves to exploit Britain's binge drinking culture.

Managers are so concerned about the consequences of the pressure to sell that they have laid bare a litany of tricks and sharp practices that will be used to maximise profits once 24-hour opening is legalised next month.

Managers for many of the big chain pubs dominating Britain's city centres are being ordered to draw up business development plans explaining how they will keep people in their pubs after 11 p.m. and offered shares of the profits if they beat sales targets. One manager told of races between bar staff to sell as many 'shots' of spirits as possible within a set time and constant pressure to 'upsell' singles to doubles.

Dave Daley, head of the National Association of Licensed House Managers, which represents Britain's thousands of pub managers, broke cover this weekend to reveal the plans. He said he was speaking out as a warning to his members not to jeopardise their livelihoods and relations with neighbouring communities by giving in to the ferocious drive to profit from bingeing.

'I have been a manager for 30 years in these superpubs and in town centres', he said. 'How we make our money is to make people binge drink: the more people drink, the more I get as a bonus. The more alcohol you sell, the more bonus you get: they give you a target to reach... We have these extra hours and companies are saying to managers "Give me your business plan, what are you going to do after 11 o'clock? If you sell x more we will give you more".'

Bonuses could be up to £20,000 a year, he said. Managers were being told that for the extra two hours they can open under the new laws, they could sell, for example, £2000 worth of extra stock and keep 10 per cent of that as a bonus.

Daley's frank admissions will be taken seriously because they represent the first indication from within the industry—which has lobbied for the relaxation of the licensing laws—that the extensions are likely to have harmful consequences.

The industry was within its rights to make a profit, Daley said, but the big chains must recognize they could not treat alcohol like any other product: 'The difference between us and other selling operations is that we are selling a drug', he said.

His comments come as an *Observer* investigation revealed the alarming ease with which customers can overindulge. A female reporter bought the equivalent of 64 units of alcohol in a Reading pub, ostensibly to share with a friend—enough alcohol to drink themselves to death—without once being challenged. The weekly recommended alcohol intake for a woman is 21 units.

James Purnell, the licensing minister, said irresponsible drinks promotions would be specifically targeted under the legislation and those found to be infringing it could lose their licences. 'Any chain using irresponsible drinking promotions to boost its profits isn't operating in the real world,' he said. 'Public opinion has hardened since the mid-1990s and the act does put people on notice that we expect to make irresponsible drinks promotions a thing of the past.'

Daley, however, said that opening later would inevitably have an impact: 'People are going to drink more, no doubt about it. Your sales are going to go up by 10–15 per cent. All this stuff about a cafe society is a lot of rubbish.'

Plans to keep drinkers in the pub after 11pm are likely to include curry nights, quiz nights or karaoke, he said, but there were concerns that pressure to maximise profits would lead to more noisy late-night entertainment which would badly affect neighbourhoods.

Mark Hastings of the British Beer and Pub Association, which represents the big managed pub chains as well as breweries, denied acting irresponsibly. Food was now a boom area for pubs and managers could meet sales targets by selling more of it, he suggested, even late at night.

'Just think of the number of people who go for a late-night curry', he said. 'As for incentives related to sales, it would be totally misinterpreting them to say this is only related to selling drink. It's about 'can you draw more customers to your pub, can you pull customers away from other pubs?' These are all ways of increasing profits.'

However, one former pub manager told the *Observer* that high-pressure sales tactics used in her pub were on orders from head office: 'Our job was to make as much money as possible—how could we do that except by selling as much alcohol as possible?'

Daley said pub managers worked on the assumption that after three or four drinks a customer was 'captured' and would stay.' (Hinscliffe and Asthana 2005)

Two days before the introduction of extended licensing the *Daily Mail* published the following report:

'Taxpayers will be subsiding huge profits for the brewers from 24-hour drinking, MPs have been warned. Local authorities say the fees they receive from pubs wanting to open longer are nowhere near enough to cover the costs of handing out late licences. Councils have had to employ hundreds of extra staff to cope with a late surge in applications—the new regime comes into force on

Thursday—as well as fight hundreds of appeals from pubs refused extended licences.' (Slack and Hickley 2005a).

Government reaction

Enter the Combat Zone

As the debate about these changes began to heat up, several news reports stated that Tony Blair and Tessa Jowell 'believed' that extending licensing hours would pave the way for a relaxed, cafe culture in England and Wales. This, it was claimed, would reduce the problems associated with Britain's notorious 'binge drinking'. It was further claimed by the DCMS that the planned changes would reduce disorder by giving the police more powers and enabling local people to 'crack down on yobbish behaviour'. No evidence has been produced to support the DCMS view. Moreover, no credible independent scientist or medical authority has apparently lent support to their claims. Over the winter of 2004/2005 the strong and wide-ranging coalition of objectors to the proposed changes prompted the government to react with a number of what appeared to be hastily conceived panic reactions. Tessa Jowell, hitherto presenting herself as an ardent advocate of liberal licensing, stated that she was opposed to 24-hour drinking and believed that pubs would not open all day (Press Association 2005).

The press and media outcry reached its first peak in late January 2005. In response to this chorus, Tessa Jowell (DCMS) and Hazel Blears (Home Office) issued a statement on January 21st. This was apparently designed to achieve two aims. The first of these was to counteract well-documented reports of Home Office opposition to DCMS licensing proposals. The second was to defuse some of the opposition. Tessa Jowell, Culture Secretary, said: 'Our current licensing laws are creaking under the strain. That's why we're reforming them-to make our towns and cities safe for all, not a free for all' (Department of Culture, Media and Sport 2005). Jowell also launched an attack on women who drank heavily.

> 'She claimed that a new breed of ladettes are drunk even before they have finished putting on their lipstick. 'They go out drunk,' she declared. Her criticism was reportedly supported by Hazel Blears.' (Slack 2005b).

Jowell stated that the Government would force pubs and clubs to pay for extra policing in trouble spots that were to be named 'alcohol disorder zones'. The latter were to be established if after an eight week period of grace, bar owners in areas beset by alcohol-fuelled disorder had not taken effective steps to reduce these problems.

An additional Government response has come in the form of 'on-the-spot' fines for bar staff who serve intoxicated patrons, and children who buy alcoholic beverages. These took effect on Monday, April 4th 2005. These fines would cost bar staff £80, while children under 16 years of age would have to pay £30 and those aged 16–17 years would have to pay £50 (Scotsman 2005b, Guardian 2005b).

Hostile media coverage of the proposed licensing changes rose to another peak in August 2005, spurred on by reports from ACPO and the Judiciary. Junior Culture Minister James Purnell attempted to defend the Government's faltering case for licensing liberalisation by claiming police support for this policy. ACPO quickly made it clear that the police did not support it. Mr Purnell acknowledged that the Government would monitor the effects of new licensing, but denied that this meant a reversal of policy was likely.

The next reaction from the Government, a predictable one, was the announcement that £5 million was to be spent on an advertising campaign to 'tackle binge drink culture'. This campaign would:

'Portray drunk behaviour as socially unacceptable and embarrassing, capitalising on disgust at images of revellers lying in gutters and vomiting in the streets.' (Hinscliffe 2005)

The effectiveness of alternative approaches to reducing alcohol problems is considered later in Chapter 7. Suffice it to note here that alcohol campaigns of this type have a dismal track record. Politically appealing because they may suggest that a government is 'acting', campaigns of this type are expensive and invariably do not change drinking habits or reduce alcohol problems. Moreover, there is real danger that a campaign along the lines suggested may simply serve to sensationalise, glamourise and add to the rebellious appeal of heavy drinking. Shock-horror tactics have long been discredited as a basis for public education.

Strikingly the Department of Health remained largely silent while the public debate raged on. One of the Department's few public contributions was a strange statement that a survey by Mintel, released in August 2005, indicated that a recent increase in alcohol consumption did not suggest that: 'People are causing harm to themselves or others from the rise in alcohol consumption' (Carvel 2005a). These remarks ignored substantial evidence, including a report from the Chief Medical Officer, on rising liver disease deaths, alcohol-related mortality in general and psychiatric illness that flatly contradicted this view. It appeared that the Department of Health, supposedly the guardian of the health of the people of England and Wales, was supporting the embattled Government's line of not wanting even the most obvious facts to influence its thinking.

Tessa Jowell reacted defiantly to a steadily mounting chorus of objections to the liberalisation of liquor licensing with an article in the *Independent on Sunday* newspaper. In this statement she reaffirmed her belief that longer bar hours were 'a necessary if not sufficient' part of a reasonable strategy to curb binge drinking. She also added that she thought that New Labour's 1997 slogan "Don't Give a XXXX for Last Orders" was 'stupid'. She also expressed the hope that a new campaign to educate young people (combined with 'decent education from parents and teachers' would help to reduce the problem (Jowell 2005a).

Additional authoritative medical voices of protest were raised in defence of public health during September 2005:

> 'Labour peer Lord Robert Winston and Professor Roger Williams, one of the country's leading liver disease consultants, said the government was failing to recognise a growing scourge of alcohol abuse. Williams, who carried out the first liver transplant in 1968 and has treated thousands of patients, said the decision to allow pubs to open for longer hours, was 'hideous.' and would lead to more alcohol-related deaths ... Williams said his main concern was the prospect of seeing more and more young lives, particularly those of young women, ruined by binge-drinking.' (Bentham and Temko 2005).

It was becoming obvious that local objections to applications for licensing extensions were being widely ignored by licensing authorities. Objections to this led the Government to announce another concession on September 16th 2005. This was reported in the *The Mail on Sunday* and the *Financial Times*. The latter carried a front page headline proclaiming: 'Backtrack on drink laws'. This was accompanied by the following report:

> 'Ministers will next week announce a significant concession over 24-hour drinking laws, in an attempt to head off a public outcry about the biggest overhaul of licensing for 900 years. The government is to write to local authorities telling them that it has bowed to their demands for an immediate rethink of the official guidance setting out how they should oversee the legislation. The Local Government Association, the body that represents councils in England and Wales, has argued that the guidelines need to be tightened to prevent an explosion of binge drinking once the new laws come into force in November. Town hall chiefs have told Tessa Jowell, the culture secretary, that the current guidance is skewed in favour of pubs, clubs and restaurants that want to open late, and that the balance should be tilted back towards local residents who object to round the clock drinking. James Purnell, the minister in charge of the licensing shake up, told the FT last night that the government wanted to be 'conciliatory,' and that the guidelines issued to local authorities and the police-would be reviewed within three months of the new regime taking effect ... Sir Sandy Bruce-Lockhart, LGA chairman, welcomed the government's plan to review this guidance. 'I have argued that the guidance is too liberalising, too strong in encouraging extended hours and too little discretion given to local authorities.'' (Newman 2005)

The Mail on Sunday reported:

> 'The last minute U-turn will also damage Tessa Jowell, who has ultimate responsibility for the late night drink legislation. However, the Culture Secretary is virtually fireproof because of her close loyalty to the Prime Minister.' (Lewis 2005a).

Another sign of Government discomfort was voiced by Charles Clarke, the Home Secretary. He complained about the manner in which the management of pub chains were behaving:

> Charles Clarke yesterday accused pub chains of trying to 'blackmail' residents who fight plans for late-night drinking. His extraordinary outburst was leapt on by critics as an admission that the Government's 24-hour drinking legislation is flawed. The Home Secretary attacked pub companies who have threatened to claim thousands of pounds in legal costs from locals who dare to appeal to magistrates ... The situation was highlighted by the case-revealed in the *Mail*—of father of two Toby Walne, of South Woodford, East London. He applied for an appeal hearing after failing to persuade councillors to stop the Laurel Pub Company opening a Hogshead pub late into the night. Lawyers for the multi-million pound firm, which owns 420 pubs, wrote to him threatening to claim thousands of pounds in legal costs if he lost his appeal.' (Hickley 2005a)

The appeal process is expensive. A single appeal is reported to have cost £30,000 (Savill 2005).

Continuing criticism of the liberalisation of licensing arrangements was casting doubt about the Prime Minister's 'Respect' agenda. This was intended to reduce public nuisance and bad behaviour. More evidence of both Governmental unease and determination in spite of the hostile reception of its plans led to another development in late September 2005:

> 'Tony Blair's willingness to embrace the law and order agenda became clear last night as Whitehall prepares to draw up powers for the police to dispense summary justice to combat antisocial behaviour and binge drinking. The new police powers include:
> Instant Asbos: much greater use of injunction-style 'interim Asbos' granted to the police without evidence or witnesses having to be heard or the defendant informed. Bans and restrictions remaining in place until a full court hearing.
> New police powers to cancel late-night extensions for rowdy pubs and clubs without having to bother the courts.
> Fixed penalty fines of £80 for drunk and disorderly behaviour. Three tickets and persistent binge drinkers will face a 'drinking banning order' barring them from pubs and clubs in a specified area for as specified time, possibly a month. Underage drinkers and those who serve them will face similar fines.' (Travis 2005b)

The reference to 'persistent binge drinkers' was curious, implying that binge drinking was invariably synonymous with illegal behaviour. In fact, it is not, even though heavy drinking and crime are strongly associated. It should be borne in mind that according to the Government's own advisors, there are 5.9

million binge drinkers in the country, many of whom may be regarded as 'persistent' (Cabinet Office 2004).

A reported rise in alcohol-related violent crime in England and Wales allegedly led government ministers to minimize its importance, claiming that the police were not 'hugely concerned' about this development. This claim was denied by the police (Hickley 2005b).

Another indication of government thinking was revealed by Ms Louise Casey, the so-called government 'Respect Czar' in October 2005. She was reported to be pressing for a ban on drinking on commuter trains, buses and trams:

> 'A rise in alcohol-related disorder on trains and buses late at night has prompted the proposal. Mersyside MPs have called for £100 fines for consuming alcohol on a local rail line where it was found that 171 reported anti-social incidents in six months were alcohol-related. The crackdown is one of several proposals arising from a meeting between Tony Blair and Casey's team at Chequers in August. Blair's attitude to the proposed ban is not known but the fact that it is being carried forward for further consideration while other ideas have been killed off suggests that it has at least his tacit support. The 'Chequers paper' a confidential list of 40 proposals discussed with the prime minister, reveals that Blair also considered introducing street breathalyser tests for binge drinkers and creating a new criminal offence of being 'dangerously drunk'.

These proposals have now been dropped. (Cracknell 2005).

The suggested alcohol ban on public transport was greeted with derision by the press. Within hours it was reported that government ministers were distancing themselves from this suggestion (White and Dodd 2005).

It was reported in November 2005 that the chief executives of Britain's main supermarkets were called in to meet Charles Clarke, the Home Secretary. Mr Clarke reportedly informed them that supermarket alcohol sales to minors were unacceptable. He threatened companies that continued to make such sales with the loss of licences (Hickman 2005).

In late November 2005 Tessa Jowell and Charles Clarke announced a £2.5 million public campaign against binge drinking. Mr Clarke acknowledged that the latter would take a long time to curb (White and Hencke 2005). In contrast to some of her earlier claims, Tessa Jowell reportedly conceded that the longer bar opening hours might be followed by more alcohol-related violent crime (Slack and Hickley 2005b). This was a remarkable admission, flatly contradicting a number of earlier statements by government ministers that they expected the opposite. Was reality beginning to break through the façade? The Government made a further surprising comment on the possible effect of licensing changes:

> 'A government admission that the new licensing laws may lead to an increase in alcohol-related offences plunged the measure into fresh controversy just 24 hours before they come into effect. As pubs, clubs and supermarkets prepared for

midnight tonight, when the new era of potential round-the-clock drinking begins, critics seized on comments by Paul Goggins who said that there may be more arrests and fixed penalty notices... 'If we spend £2.5 m increasing the strength of enforcement and funding police to do it, it is likely that the number of arrests and fixed penalty notices will go up', the minister said.' (Travis, Muir and Cowan 2005)

It was also announced that the impact of new licensing laws would be assessed by 'scrutiny councils' in Birmingham, Blackpool, Brighton, Bristol, Cardiff, Havering, Manchester, Newcastle upon Tyne, Nottingham, and Taunton Deane (Travis, Muir and Cowan 2005).

On November 23rd, 2005, just hours before the new licensing hours came into force the *Daily Mirror* published the following comment by Tessa Jowell:

'Britain has a drink problem. As a nation we drink too much, too fast. The cost to the NHS and to our quality of life has been captured a thousand times on CCTC cameras.

For nearly a century, the Government has effectively created a national curfew with all pubs shut by 11pm. But this has only made matters worse.

Drinkers compete to empty their glasses before last orders, then get chucked out at the same time to fight (literally) for taxis and food.

The result? Nearly half of all incidents of violence and disorder happen between 11pm and midnight on Friday and Saturday nights.

All that changes with the new licensing laws. Publicans can stay open longer if they satisfy police, residents and the council that they won't cause trouble.

Revellers will also have more freedom but can be fined on the spot or arrested if they misbehave.

There is a simple logic to this new law. Adults should be trusted to make their own decisions about when and how they have a night out. But yobbish behaviour will be punished hard and swift. The police have more powers to tackle disorder, and I want them to use everyone. This approach is paying off in central Birmingham. In the busy Broad Street area, pubs and clubs have stopped irresponsible drinks promotions that just aim to get people drunk quickly. Venues also pay for extra policing, resulting in a massive 25 per cent reduction in violent crime last year.

But Britain's binge culture is too deep-seated to be changed with just one law. There's much more to do. We must ensure the drinks industry is responsible.

So today's changes aren't the solution. But they are an important start. At least we've got our priorities right: zero-tolerance for the yobbish minority and freedom for the adult who just wants a quiet night out.' (Jowell 2005b).

Reaction to the Government's response

Political response

The Licensing Act had received Parliamentary approval with only muted objections. In spite of this, political alarm mounted as the public debate gathered pace in late 2004 and during 2005. Politicians from all three major political parties added their voices in protest against the planned liberalisation of licensing hours. The Conservative party and the Liberal Democrats called for delay or modification of the plan. Both parties called for the Government to postpone plans to extend bar opening hours (Scotsman 2005b). Even Labour Party members of Parliament, including former Government ministers David Blunkett and Frank Dobson, made it clear that they believed the proposed measures would increase alcohol-related problems. The House of Commons (all-party) Home Affairs Committee produced a report, *Anti-Social Behaviour*, that was published in early April 2005. This document called for the banning of cheap drink promotions in public houses and clubs. Moreover, this committee recommended a levy on licensees to cover the costs of policing and other services needed to respond to alcohol-related disorder and other allied problems (House of Commons Home Affairs Committee 2005). The introduction of on-the-spot fines for bar staff serving drunken patrons and for under-age alcohol buyers were criticised by the (Conservative) Shadow Home Secretary as a 'patchwork response which would not solve the problem of alcohol-fuelled yobbery in Britain's town and city centres' (Scotsman 2005b). During August 2005 David Davis, the Shadow Home Secretary, called for licensing changes to be tested out in a few select areas (White 2005).

Mark Oaten, the Liberal Democrat Shadow Home Secretary was quoted in the *Daily Mail* on January 12th 2005 as follows: 'When the problem is running out of control in our town centres, extending drinking hours to 24 hours a day is madness.' By the summer of 2005 Conservative Leader Michael Howard was calling for the new licensing arrangements to be put on hold until binge drinking had been curbed. The Liberal Democrats shared this view.

During August 2005 the *Times* reported that Government ministers were concerned that there might be back-bench revolt in support of opposition party demands for compromise on new drinking laws. It was also reported that the Liberal Democrats and Conservatives were planning a late attempt to moderate the impending new licensing laws: 'They will use a little known parliamentary process called "praying" in an attempt to wring concessions from the Government.' It was also reported that there would be further opposition to the licensing changes from within the House of Lords. It was speculated that this opposition would be forced to back down as they had done early in 2005 in relation to an unpopular plan to establish a new network of Las Vegas-style casinos. (Bennett *et al.* 2005, Brown and Woolf 2005).

Mark Oaten elaborated the Liberal Democrat position in September 2005:

> '. . . the Liberal Democrats in principle support the liberalisation of the licensing laws. We believe that with the right control and support mechanisms in place, flexible licensing hours could reduce the problems caused by binge drinking and

alcohol-related violence. However, despite the Government's good intentions, we are concerned that the current legislation doesn't include adequate safeguards and for this reason we voted against the Bill at its 2nd and 3rd readings.

Our understanding is that despite media fears, the current data and economics of the industry makes so called '24 hour drinking' extremely unlikely. There are still many outstanding issues, like who will pay for the extra policing required in town centres. I have called for a levy on the large drinking establishments to tackle potential havoc in city centres and to prevent the burden falling on local taxpayers.

Obviously binge drinking also remains a problem and I am concerned that the Government is only just getting to grips with the problems associated with binge drinking. I have argued that the liberalisation of licensing laws should be post-poned until measures to prevent binge drinking have been put in place and shown to be effective. Proposals like 'Alcohol Disorder Zones' and action to fine bar staff who serve drunken customers should have been trialled before the extended hours legislation comes into effect.

It is clear that the Government have mishandled the introduction of a prom-ising policy and that there are a number of shortcomings with the current provisions. The Liberal Democrats argue the extension of hours should be delayed until proper safeguards are in place. (Oaten 2005)

Don Foster, the Liberal Democrat Shadow Culture Secretary, criticized a Government decision to exempt nightclubs from contributing to the costs of policing drunkenness (Foster 2005a). Conversations with several Labour MPs revealed that they were unhappy about this legislation, but in some cases were nervous about saying this publicly. Some on the Labour side did object publicly. These included Labour peer Lord Simon of Highbury who objected to his local pub extending its hours (Delgado 2005). During September 2005 it was reported that even a number of cabinet ministers were becoming concerned:

'One senior Minister told *The Mail on Sunday:* 'I witnessed shocking scenes when I left the cinema at the same time as the pubs were closing'. Other ministers have told of similar behaviour at a time when the Government is trying to bring in new measures to foster respect and responsibility in our society. Against this back-ground we cannot be seen to be also advocating drunkenness and thuggery.' (Lewis 2005a).

Liberal Democrat concerns about Government policy were further voiced in a letter to the *Guardian* by Don Foster:

'Tessa Jowell's determination to press ahead with the Licensing Act despite the mounting public concern is complete folly... She claims the act will benefit the 'responsible majority,' yet they don't want it. They want excessive drinking under control before making alcohol more available. They know that research shows that in countries where serious alcohol-related social problems exist, longer licensing hours made these problems worse, not better.

Jowell talks of the benefits of tougher police powers. Yet we don't even use existing ones. While it's already illegal to sell alcohol to someone who is drunk, nationwide there are fewer than a dozen prosecutions each year. Where new police powers could help, then they can be added to the violent-crime reduction bill currently before parliament.' (Foster 2005b)

In October 2005 confirmation was given that there would be a final attempt by opposition parties to block the licensing liberalisation coming into effect:

The Conservatives are to use an obscure parliamentary procedure in a last-ditch attempt to block the 24-hour drinking laws due to be introduced next month. Theresa May, the Tory culture spokesman, will tomorrow lodge a motion for a procedure known as 'praying against a statutory instrument'. This will have the effect of forcing another Commons vote on the Licensing Act in the next few weeks. The Conservatives and Liberal Democrats will unite to vote against the act and Tory whips claim they have the support of a growing number of Labour backbenchers. Many Labour MPs have been alarmed by criticism from police, doctors and constituents. Frank Dobson, a former Labour Health Secretary, said: 'The whole thing is geared towards extending licensing laws. The bias of the thing is harmful. The assumption that spreading closing times will reduce the impact (of binge drinking) is claptrap. The Tories are using the praying device against an order setting a date for the new act to take effect'. The order, in the form of a statutory instrument, would normally pass without a hitch. May said: 'These laws are deeply unpopular and potentially disastrous. This is our final opportunity to force the government to abandon its plans'. The Tories are also planning to use the Lords to block the act. Lord Winston, the fertility specialist and Labour peer said: 'Like most of the medical profession I associate alcohol with serious problems, particularly aggression. This is a poten-tially risky step. My instinct is that I could not support this bill'. (Newell and Watt 2005)

The Government reacted to the threat posed by this latest action in the form of a letter to MPs by James Purnell, minister in the DCMS. This letter warned that a delay in the introduction of the planned licensing arrangements would cause chaos. Remarkably this letter was supported by the Association of Chief Police Officers.

He pointed out in his letter that a delay 'would cause administrative chaos over Christmas and the New Year as more than 100,000 premises would need to apply for and pay for over 400,000 special permissions to sell alcohol late just to cover Christmas events during the festive period. This would threaten the livelihood of many businesses'. He also told the *Guardian* 'It's a shame that the Conservatives and LibDems want to play politics with the act in Westminster this autumn. But it flies in the face of what is happening on the ground and the express wishes of ACPO, who don't want a delay'. (Wintour 2005a)

A rise in violent crime prompted both Conservative and Liberal Democrat spokesmen (Edward Gardner and Mark Oaten) to repeat appeals to the government to defer the planned licensing liberalisation (Travis 2005a).

The Home Secretary Charles Clarke, announced at a meeting described as a 'booze summit' on October 19th that supermarkets would be ordered to 'crack down' on selling alcohol to minors. It was reported that this move was in response to the widespread criticism of the planned liberalisation of the licensing laws (Worthington 2005).

> 'Many are worried about the government allowing pubs to serve drink into the early hours of the morning, and reports that pressure is being put on bar staff to serve more and more alcohol to customers are a very real concern," said Shadow Culture Secretary Theresa May.' (Hinscliffe and Asthana 2005).

Licensing reform was again debated in the House of Commons on October 24th, 2004:

> '**Mrs Theresa May (Maidenhead) (Con):** I beg to move, that this House notes the growing public concern that the Licensing Act 2003 will increase levels of violent crime and anti-social behaviour; observes that the cost to the taxpayer of rising alcohol-fuelled crime and disorder is already £12 billion a year; objects to the presumption in favour of late-night drinking irrespective of the views of local residents and local representatives; disapproves of the disproportionate burden of administration and increased costs for village halls, sports clubs and community centres; calls for local councils to have greater discretion to take into account the interests of their local community; and calls on the Government to cancel the full commencement of the Act and overhaul the primary legislation.
>
> It is a matter of record that, since the Committee stage of the Licensing Bill, my party has consistently raised our concerns about the implications of the Government's proposal to introduce extended licensing hours. Both in Committee and since, we have argued that the drinking culture in the UK—in particular, the culture of binge drinking and the explosion of alcohol-fuelled violence and anti-social behaviour—has made the Government's plans dangerous and foolhardy.
>
> Ministers offered us a number of reassurances in Committee. At the same time as promising that Labour could not give a XXXX for drinking-up time, the Prime Minister was also pledging: 'We will tackle the unacceptable level of anti-social behaviour and crime on our streets. Our 'zero tolerance' approach will ensure that petty criminality among young offenders is seriously addressed.'
>
> The reality on our streets is very different. There are now 1 million violent crimes a year and, in the three months to June, police recorded 318,200 violent crimes—up 6 per cent on the same period last year. A particularly worrying statistic is that half the violence is due to binge drinking.

... Figures out last week showed violent crime up by 6 per cent. on the same period last year. The Secretary of State has already referred to the link between binge drinking and violent crime, so does she not accept that the new licensing hours will simply make the problem worse?

Ms Tessa Jowell: No, I certainly do not. The Association of Chief Police Officers wants the Act to be implemented on time, as do local authorities. They recognise something that seems to have escaped the Right Hon. Lady for many weeks—the police need those new powers to tackle alcohol-related crime. In her constant opportunistic opposition she is in effect voting against the voices in the police and local government saying that we need those powers to make a serious attack on alcohol-related crime.

Mrs May: I suggest that the Secretary of State listen more carefully to the question in future. I did not ask about the Licensing Law and the new powers; I asked about the new licensing hours. Senior police officers have made it clear that new powers are welcome but that extended licensing hours are not. A Scotland Yard report predicts an 'increase in the number of investigations of drink-related crimes, such as rape, assault, homicide and domestic violence.' The chief constable of North Yorkshire said that longer hours would lead to: 'increased criminality, drink-driving, road casualties and antisocial behaviour.' The licensing spokesman for the Association of Chief Police Officers said: 'People are going to drink more because of longer hours and there will be lots more crime and disorder.'

Why are the Government ignoring them?

Tessa Jowell: Some of the crimes that people commit while under the influence of alcohol are hideous. There is no dispute in the House about that, but I would not want the Right Hon. Lady to think that this was a decision that was reached lightly. The Government are determined to push ahead with the implementation of the Licensing Act, because we can provide protection to innocent victims by giving the police powers to take effective action. She used a pick-and-mix strategy to find a chief constable who agrees with her, but the president of ACPO has made it quite clear that the police do not have any objection to flexible hours per se. We have worked closely with the police to meet their concerns. We are going to implement the legislation on 24 November and many people will be saved from attack, assault and injury as a result.' (Hansard October 24th 2005)

Two more last minute attempts were made in Parliament to block the imminent introduction of extended liquor licensing hours. The House of Lords voted to delay the introduction of the new licensing arrangements on November 14th. Liberal democrat peer Lord McNally commented in the debate on that day:

'Another of the Government's main justifications for the new licensing law was to vary closing hours and curb drunken violence on the streets at weekends. However, in a British Beer and Pub Association poll, 90 per cent of its 30,000 members had only applied for an extra one or two hours' opening time, with the majority applying to close at midnight. Figures like those suggest that midnight will become

the new chucking-out time. Closing times will be deferred as a opposed to stag-
gered, and we have the situation where, as Chris Allsion, lead officer on licensing at
the Association of Chief Police Officers has warned: 'People will have drunk more
and are more likely to get into fights'. (Liberal Democrats Online 2005).

The following day, November 15th, a Conservative-led motion to delay the
liberalization was defeated in the House of Commons by a government
majority of 74 votes. Speaking in this debate the Shadow Culture Secretary,
Theresa May, declared that the new licensing plans were 'in the last chance
saloon'. She described the changes as reckless and likely to add to current levels
of violence and disorder. Licensing Minister James Purnell repeated his view
(on the Radio Four Today programme) that the changes were intended to treat
people as grown ups (Slack and Hickley 2005b). In late November 2005,
Theresa May accused the Deputy Prime Minister, John Prescott, of covering
up evidence on the impact of heavy drinking. This charge was prompted by a
report that Mr Prescott had instructed local authorities to discontinue collat-
ing statistics on alcohol-related crimes. Mr Prescott's department denied this
allegation (Lewis 2005b).

Admissions by government ministers that licensing changes might lead to a
higher levels of alcohol-related crime because of better enforcement were
criticized by both Conservative and Liberal Democrat representatives. Conservative Theresa May commented:

> 'According to Mr Purnell's logic, the drunker and more violent people get on
> Thursday night, the better job he will have done.' (Travis, Muir and Cowan 2005)

Liberal Democrat Mark Foster remarked: 'This is like a bad episode of Yes
Minister. It's pure double-speak'. (Hickley and Mills 2005)

The Liberal Democrats released figures indicating that alcohol-related crime
had increased by 20% in the past two years:

> 'Don Foster, their spokesman, said there were already 1,000 offences a week
> connected to alcohol-fuelled violence and increasing the availability of alcohol
> would make matters worse.' (Johnston 2005)

The Police

The Government's January 21st statement was initially welcomed by Mr Chris
Fox, President of the Association of Chief Police Officers (ACPO). Even so a
more considered and far less positive ACPO comment was issued in March
2005. The Government proposals were described by ACPO as 'a short term fix'.
An ACPO view was described in the *Observer* newspaper:

> 'The document highlights the police's fear that the creation of alcohol disorder
> zones (ADZs), the government's latest response to concerns about the links

between longer hours and yob behaviour, would cost the taxpayer and see officers spending more time in court rather than crime fighting... 'We're fundamentally missing the issue here. Extending the licensing hours does not mean people are going to stop drinking 14 pints of lager, choose French wine, become fluent in French and sit in a pavement café; what they are going to do is have 16 pints instead.' Said Chris Allison, a commander with the Metropolitan Police who coordinates ACPO's response on licensing issues... ACPO has called for the government to develop a multi-pronged approach to curbing drink-related problems, which would include a plan for drinks companies to pay for extra policing. Without such an approach, ACPO insisted, problems thrown up by Britain's drinking culture cannot be solved." (Doward 2005).

ACPO warned the Government again in August 2005 that liberalising liquor licensing would 'turn many town and city centres into the local equivalent of drink-fuelled Mediterranean hotspots' (White 2005). It should be noted that the police were not agreeing with the Government's hope that the new arrangements would usher in a utopian era of relaxed café wine drinking. On the contrary, police chiefs made it clear that they feared British urban areas would witness the notorious excesses associated with popular holiday destinations such as Faliraki and Ibiza. The police also noted that:

> 'There is a strong link between the increase in disorder and the explosion of late night premises... The assertion that 11pm closing leads to binge drinking is simply not supported by the evidence.'

Since early 2005 substantial and growing police opinion has been hostile to plans to extend bar opening hours. Government ministers have consistently ignored this advice while urging people to heed police views on countering terrorism. The Police Federation, representing 138,000 officers warned that extended bar opening hours would strain police resources. This would mean that more police time would be spent dealing with disorder after later closing and reduce the police available for daytime duties (Sparrow 2005). Further objections to the proposed liberalisation of liquor licensing came from the British Transport Police (BTP) (2005). Launching the annual report of this organization, the Chief Constable, Ian Johnston, reported that the BTP feared that the new licensing hours would necessitate extra police patrols to deal with an upsurge of crimes in the early hours of the morning, he also noted that alcohol-related crime had risen by almost a third in the previous year (Bowcott 2005).

Another disturbing newspaper report noted that:

> 'Police are powerless to block thousands of pubs and bars from extending their opening hours because they cannot link them to violent crime, senior officers have told the *Times*.

A *Times* survey has found that police in cities and urban areas throughout England and Wales have lodged a tiny number of objections to plans by pubs to open longer.

In most areas fewer than 5 per cent of applications have prompted representations or objections from the police...

Commander Chris Allison of the Association of Chief Police Officers, said:

'We are seeing hundreds of licensed premises applying for an extra hour during the week and two at weekends. People are going to drink more because of longer hours and there will be lots more crime and disorder.' (Ford *et al.* 2005)

An additional alarming warning note was sounded by the Metropolitan Police:

'Rapes and murders are expected to soar as a result of 24-hour drinking, according to a confidential Scotland Yard study. It predicts that other violent crimes, including domestic violence, will rise along with drink-driving when round-the-clock opening hours are introduced in November... In a 30-page internal report, the Metropolitan Police's Clubs and Vice Unit says that the new licensing laws will result in a massive drain on police resources. It calls for the force's riot squad to be put on 24-hour standby to cope with the surge in offences. It also warns that the number of police on the streets will fall sharply as officers spend more time in police stations processing drunks being held for public order offences and assaults. Such offenders can take five times longer to process than suspects who are sober. There may also be a shortage of cells.' (Wright 2005)

It was reported during November 2005 that the police were concerned that the proposed licensing changes would simply create a new, later, bar closing time. This comment followed the revelation that many licensees were planning to adopt midnight as their closing time:

'The prospect of near-simultaneous closing for most pubs when the law comes into force on November 24th has alarmed police. Chris Allison lead officer on licensing at the Association of Chief Police Officers (ACPO) said forces across the country had contacted him with concerns about the simultaneous closing time falling an hour later than at present. 'People will have drunk more and are likely to get into fights', he said. "What we will have to deal with is large number of people coming on to the streets at the same time, fighting for services that may not be there".' (Iredale 2005)

Just a few days before the introduction of the extended opening hours the police reacted angrily to the disclosure that they were not being given new enforcement powers as soon as the longer bar hours were introduced. It had been anticipated that they would be able to set up alcohol disorder zones and ban chronic trouble makers from town and city centres from November 24th 2005. In fact, it emerged that the Violent Crime Reduction Bill was unlikely to take effect until the summer of 2006 (Slack 2005c). Ms Jan Berry, chair of the

Police Federation commented as follows just before the new licensing laws came into force:

> 'Whether extending licensing hours will deliver responsible drinking, we remain to be convinced... If we find in a few months' time, that police are facing more violence because of excess alcohol, then we will need to go back to the government and ask them to reverse the decision.' (Travis, Muir and Cowan 2005)

Other voices

Ms Srabani Sen, Chief Executive of Alcohol Concern said: 'We applaud many of the steps taken by this government to tackle the nation's binge drinking problem, but the proposals today have not fixed the fundamental flaws of the Licensing Act'. (Form Briefs 2005, Travis 2005c). A report by the investment bank Goldman Sachs has estimated that extended opening hours will boost alcohol sales by £500 million (Ungoed-Thomas and Swinford 2005). Industry representatives denied that such big profits were expected (Slack 2005c). A few days before the new opening hours were due to take effect, the Chartered Institute for Environmental Health warned that the new arrangements would impose a big strain on their already overstretched resources and that public health would be put at risk:

> 'The 10,500 environmental health officers will be in the front line against the predicted rise in drink-related problems when pubs and clubs are allowed to stay open longer... Along with the police, the officers will be monitoring disturbances outside problem pubs and reviewing licences.' (Doward *et al.* 2005).

Criticism of the plan to extend bar opening hours came from a surprising source, Tony Booth, the Prime Minister's father-in-law:

> 'Longer licensing hours won't suddenly turn us into a nation of Mediterranean sophisticates happy to make a small glass of red wine last an hour or two at some pavement café... In this country we don't drink that way. We drink in a more primitive, frightening, Anglo-Saxon way. We drink to get drunk.' (Daily Mail 2005b)

The judiciary

It was revealed that judges in England and Wales had issued a remarkable statement of concern about the planned liberalisation of licensing hours on August 10th. A report by the Council of Her Majesty's Circuit Judges warned the Home Office that the proposed changes would lead to increase in alcohol-related violence, rape and other serious crimes. This report stated:

> 'We regard it as wishful thinking to suppose that the introduction of the Licensing Act will bring about the cultural change which the Government envisages.' (Ford and Tendler 2005)

Judge Charles Harris expressed his personal concern in the following strong terms:

> 'It is very rare for any of these offences of violence to be committed by someone who has not been drinking. Sometimes the quantity of alcohol is simply beyond belief. A gallon is common, 12 pints by no means rare. Often these quantities of beer are diluted by various additions of spirits. It is becoming common, too, for cocaine to be taken as well. It is not just the illiterate and inarticulate underclass which does this, quite bright people in well-paid jobs (with a surprising number of women). Their whole idea of fun is to get as drunk as possible in bars where this can be done as easily as possible. .... The more there is to drink, and the more time to drink it, they will keep drinking. If it were not for the widespread availability of alcohol I believe crimes of violence would be at very modest levels indeed ... The situation is already grave, if not grotesque, and to facilitate this by making drinking facilities more widely available is close to lunacy. It simply means that our town and city centres are abandoned every night to tribes of pugnacious, drunk, noisy, vomiting louts.' (Harris 2005)

The beverage alcohol industry

The beverage alcohol industry is not monolithic. The alcohol producers appear to have said little in public about this controversy. Even so, Government proposals (on January 21st 2005) to charge bar owners for the costs of extra policing following the introduction of extended hours has been met with hostility by the British Beer and Pub Association. In addition, Mr Tim Martin

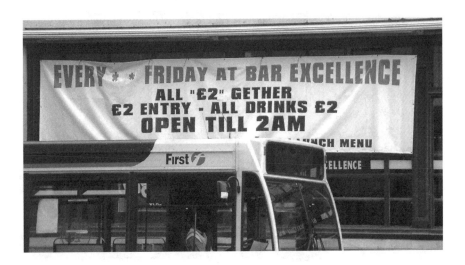

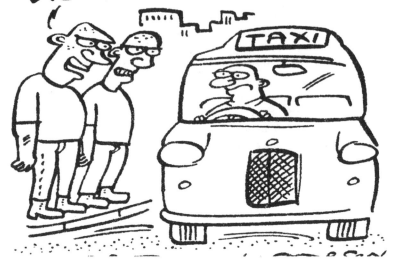

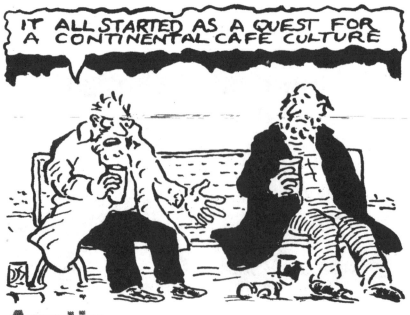

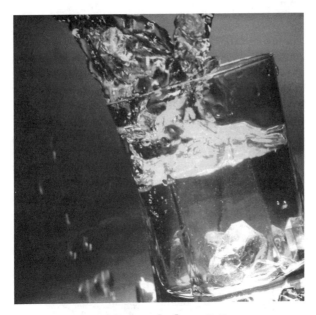

Double Up
for half the price

available on all spirits

Austin

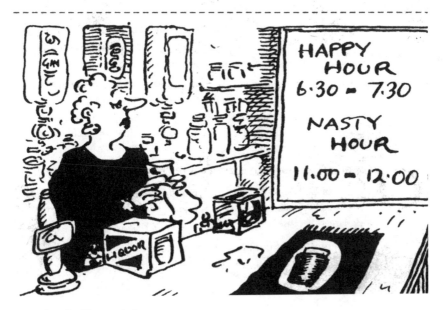

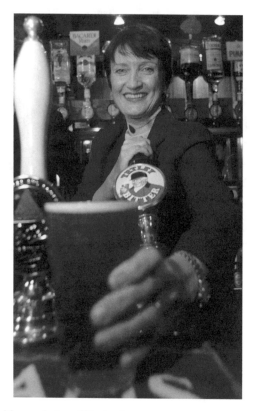

Tessa Jowell (with permission of Revters).

of J.D. Wetherspoons, a company owning 650 bars, described the Home Office officials responsible for the move towards 24-hour pub opening as 'morons'. He also noted; 'It was never an idea that emerged from pubs'. (Slack 2005e, p.5). The head of Britain's biggest family brewery has also reportedly criticized government plans:

'James Arkell... fears competition will force many pubs out of business as they open later in a bid to 'outdo' each other... he accused the government of washing its hands of the binge drinking crisis by offloading responsibility on to local councils.' (Chapman 2005)

A survey of pub landlords conducted for the BBC found:

'no appetite for 24 hour opening... None of the publicans responding to the BBC survey said they planned to apply for licenses allowing them to open round the clock, largely because it would not be financially viable' (Observer 2005).

An interim indication of publicans' response to the opportunity to apply for longer opening hours emerged on March 18th, 2005. The BBC reported that nobody had applied for an all-day licence, and very few had applied for even modest extensions of their opening hours:

> 'Landlords appear to be concerned over attention given to rowdy, anti-social behaviour by drinkers in city centres... Even in areas with no history of trouble, licensees appear worried that applications would trigger vocal objections. They are concerned objections would come not only from neighbours but also from councillors who the government has made responsible for regulating the industry... the plans have caused controversy and are opposed by some police chiefs and medics who are worried about binge drinking.' (BBC 2005)

The British Beer and Pub Association (BBPA) announced an initiative on May 23rd 2005. It called for a ban on happy hours and other cheap drinks promotions in its 32,000 bars. These account for approximately 54% of the UK's 59,000 pubs. Mr Mark Hastings of the BBPA commented:

> 'Offers like pay £10 at the door and all drinks are free, drinking games and schemes that encourage people to drink too much too quickly have no place in our sector and we are determined to stamp them out. With the backing of the Government, the Police and the Licensing authorities across the UK we aim to ensure that all pubs operate to these standards of corporate and communal social responsibility.'

This statement demonstrated that concern about the opposition to liberalizing licensing arrangements was being taken seriously by a substantial sector of the alcohol selling industry. The hitherto taboo subject of voluntary price control even reared its head. In October 2004 the Yates Group had publicly undertaken not to sell beer at less than £1.25 a pint in its 1309 pubs. It was also reported in May 2005 that Tessa Jowell favoured price controls to prevent alcohol being sold too cheaply in bars.

During July 2005 it was announced that three huge supermarket chains, Asda, Sainsbury's and Tesco, had applied for licences to sell alcoholic drinks round-the-clock. This was a significant development since such stores sell alcohol at lower prices than pubs or clubs. It was reported in August 2005 that 2000 supermarkets were planning to sell alcoholic drinks until late at night. In addition, at least 900 of these were likely to sell alcohol 24 hours each day. Steve Green, Chief Constable of Nottinghamshire, was reported to have stated:

> 'There is potential for people to pile out of nightclubs, grab more alcohol and cause mayhem on their streets or the local park because of the new licensing regulations.' (Hickley 2005c)

It was reported in August 2005 that:

> 'At least 130,000 pubs, clubs and restaurants are planning to extend their opening hours to midnight during the week and up to 2am at weekends, under proposals to

relax the licensing laws from November. About two-thirds of licensed premises have applied for extended opening. With two weeks to go before the deadline for members of the public to register any opposition with local authorities, there have been few protests and late opening is expected to become the norm in most parts of England and Wales.' (Carvel 2005a)

Urbium, owner of the Tiger group of late-night bars, disputed Westminster City Council's ban on letting children into its premises. Oliver (2005b) reported that other pub chains were taking similar action:

'The pub and bar chains have found a loophole in the Licensing Act that will allow young children in. This states that pubs can apply for a license allowing under 16s to enter the premises and be served with a non alcoholic drink-provided they are accompanied by an 'adult.' There is no curfew limiting how late a child can remain, so even those not in their teens could remain all night... Last night, a senior London police officer closely involved with licensing policy said 'We are seriously concerned that the new law will make it harder for us to keep under age children out of pubs'.'

By November 2005 it was reported that:

'At least 700 pubs, clubs and supermarkets have been granted 24-hour licenses to serve alcohol, destroying Labour's claim that there would be no more than a handful.'

It was also reported that Government ministers had written to chief constables providing them with advice on how to deal with a possible surge in alcohol-related violence following the arrival of longer bar hours (Slack 2005d).

The findings of a poll carried out for the BBC's 24 Hour News service were released on November 23rd 2005:

'About one-third of all the pubs, clubs and shops in England and Wales licensed to sell alcohol are to get longer opening hours, the BBC research suggests. New licensing laws which could allow 24-hour drinking in some areas come into force at midnight. According to the research 60,326 outlets will be allowed to sell alcohol for longer than they do now. But so far only a fraction—359 pubs and clubs—will get 24-hour licences.' (BBC News Online 2005 h).

Another subject that became controversial during 2005 was the Government's plan to ban smoking in pubs in England. It emerged that this ban might not include bars that did not serve food. The British Medical Association objected to this exemption, pointing out that a disproportionate number of such bars were in working class areas, where smoking and its related ills were most widespread. The Government plan would serve to perpetuate or increase major social inequalities in health. The British Beer and Pub Association reported that over a third of pubs might stop serving food to evade the smoking ban (Guardian 2005c). If true, this would be a retrograde step, taking many bars back to the age of bars being places where people go simply to smoke and drink. This would move British pubs even further away from the idealised continental café-bar, where food is so important. Continued smoking in bars would also be grim news for bar staff. The latter already have high lung cancer mortality rates. Their alcohol-related liver cirrhosis rates are also high. It should be noted that smoking in pubs was banned in the Republic of Ireland in March 2004. This move has been very popular and has achieved a very high level of compliance. A smoking ban in bars was introduced in Scotland in March 2006. In addition, the Welsh Assembly is seeking powers to introduce a wide-ranging ban on smoking in public places. Opinion polls show that such a ban has a high and increasing, level of support (Doward and Asthana 2005). In October 2005 it was announced that Tony Blair had 'given way' and performed a U-turn on his previous opposition to a complete ban on smoking in bars in England (Hinscliffe and Doward 2005, p.1). It was also reported that this apparent change of heart was influenced by events related to the liberalisation of bar opening hours:

'Mr Blair wants to avoid a repeat of the kind of backlash provoked by the government's once popular plan to relax the licensing laws.' (Wintour 2005b, p.7).

Pressure for an English smoking ban increased in October 2005 when it was announced that such a ban would be introduced in Northern Ireland, with effect from 2007. The proposed Northern Ireland restrictions would cover all bars and enclosed public places (Chrisafis and Carvel 2005). Later in October 2005 it was reported that there was a 'cabinet war' over the smoking ban and that Culture Secretary Tessa Jowell was not only in favour of a full ban, but was 'leading a revolt' to support it (Elliott 2005). This stance was in striking contrast to Ms Jowell's continued support for extending bar opening hours. A reportedly heated Cabinet argument about the proposed ban led to a 'compromise' proposal in the Health Bill in late October 2005. This stated that smoking would be banned in all workplaces, in England, including restaurants and pubs selling food, from 2007.

The decision to exempt mainly working-class pubs that did not serve food was also denounced as a missed opportunity by the British Medical Association and the anti-smoking pressure group ASH (Wintour 2005c). Mr Sam Galbraith, Scotland's former Health Minister, commented on the compromise plan for English pubs on the BBC Radio's Today programme on October 29th by expressing the view that it would be 'just a stage towards a total ban'. He also criticised the compromise arrangement for being:

'... patronising towards poorer people because places that will allow smoking will generally be in disadvantaged areas... It is the equivalent of getting a new vaccine for avian flu but saying we are only going to give it to the middle class but you in the working class, in the poorer areas, you're not going to get it because your life is not quite worth so much.' (BBC News Online 2005b)

MPs voted for a total ban on smoking in English pubs on February 14th, 2006.

Public opinion

A survey of Scottish opinion on liquor licensing issues was carried out in 2002. This revealed that 56% of adults reported that the existing number of licensed premises (such as pubs, off-licences and supermarkets) was 'about right'. Sixty two per cent reported that they believed current bar opening hours were also 'about right'. In addition, 21% favoured extending the current hours and 13% favoured reducing them. Nearly a quarter of those surveyed reported that they believed extending bar opening hours would reduce binge drinking (Scottish Executive 2002).

The lobby group the Campaign for Real Ale (CAMRA) reported on a survey on licensing hours in early 2003. This study showed that 75% of those questioned who expressed a view, supported publicans' right to open whenever they pleased, provided 'the local community is protected from excessive noise and nuisance... 60% of adults believe that there would be less disorder in town centres if pub closing times varied and 67% think adults should be treated as adults and have the opportunity to drink in pubs at any time they chose' (Campaign for Real Ale 2003).

It is not surprising, in view of the widespread criticisms that have been expressed during the winter of 2004/2005 that public opinion to the proposed liberalisation changed to be mainly hostile. This was confirmed by an ICM poll carried out for the BBC's Breakfast programme on January 24th, 2005. The poll showed that:

'62% believed that the new licensing laws would make the country a worse place, as against 26% who thought it would be better. An even higher proportion— 67%—thought that the new legislation would lead to an increase in anti-social behaviour compared with just 22% who thought that disorder on the streets would decline. Opinions were, however, divided on the issue of whether the existing 11pm closing time was out of date—with 46% saying it was against and 50% who thought it was not.' (BBC News Online 2005c)

The following day another poll published by the *Guardian* indicated that:

'Public support for the government's plans to reform the licensing laws has turned into outright majority opposition in only three months, according to the results of this month's Guardian/ICM poll. The survey shows that the campaign against liberalising drinking laws in England and Wales has provoked one of the sharpest swings in public opinion in recent history... In October (2004) the Guardian/ICM poll showed a clear 57% majority for the government's move to relax the drinking laws to allow pubs to stagger their closing times, with only 37% saying they disapproved. But this month's survey shows that the level of approval has fallen to only 39% and opposition has risen sharply to 53%. Only one group of voters had retained their staunch support for the measure—the 64% of 18 to 24-year-olds who presumable hope to take advantage of the extended hours. In all other age groups support has turned into opposition.' (Travis 2005d)

During March 2005 BBC Wales released the findings of a poll of 512 people aged 16 years and over in Wales. This showed that 59% (weighted percentage) believed that extending licensing hours would have an adverse effect (BBC Wales 2005). A strange episode occurred in July 2005. In an after dinner speech to police chiefs, the Head of the Home Office's Anti-Social Behaviour Unit, Louise Casey, reportedly mocked the Government campaign against binge drinking. She described official messages about binge drinking as 'nonsense'. Moreover, she was alleged to have claimed that Government Ministers might perform more effectively if 'they turn up in the morning pissed'. The *Daily Mail* newspaper claimed that Home Office officials walked out of the dinner after hearing these strange remarks. (BBC News Online 2005j).

The findings of another opinion survey were released in August 2005. This indicated that:

'Two thirds of adults aged over 18 thought it was reasonable for closing time in pubs and bars to be midnight or later... Just under a third (32%) of GB adults think the current closing time of 11pm is acceptable for pubs and bars. 30% think closing time should be extended to midnight. A further 34% think closing time should be after midnight (including 12% who back 24 hour opening). In all, almost two-thirds (64%) think closing time from midnight onwards is reason-able.' Curiously, the same survey concluded that most adults did not believe that extended licensing would have beneficial effects. Roughly three-quarters of those surveyed indicated that extending licensing would lead to an increase in anti-social behaviour, alcohol-related illness and violence. Finally, 82% reported that longer opening hours would generate more profits for the drinks industry.' (British Market Research Bureau 2005).

The findings of another opinion poll were reported in the *Times* in September 2005. This revealed that 34% of those surveyed supported the planned licensing changes, but 62% were opposed to them. Moreover, 55% of those surveyed reported that flexible bar opening times would increase public disorder, noise and nuisance. A total of 42% disagreed with this view (Times 2005).

An interesting example of public response to proposed licensing extensions in three local pubs was provided by a public meeting that took place in July 2005 in a village in South Gloucestershire. Over 150 people attended this event. With the exception of a single licensee who was applying to keep his pub open late at night, all of those who spoke at this gathering were strongly opposed to any extension of the opening hours of their local pubs. These individuals represented a wide range of ages and backgrounds. They included a publican, police officers, retired people, labourers, and professionals. Many stated that the level of alcohol-related nuisance and property damage after pub closing time was already excessive and that they had suffered badly from this. A police officer admitted that the police simply lacked the resources to record, let alone respond to, many complaints related to such nuisance. It was also alleged that two of the three local pubs were known noisy trouble spots and that staff at one establishment routinely served alcohol to underage teenagers and to people who were obviously drunk. This village was not exceptional and the statements made at this meeting gave a good indication of the way in which local communities are affected by the harmful effects of noisy or badly behaved drinkers. Shortly after this meeting licensing authorities in South Gloucestershire granted extended licences to two of these pubs in spite of a considerable number of objections. This decision meant that for the first time this small village would have late night drinking establishments guarded by 'bouncers'. These extensions were permitted even though it had been made clear that villagers neither needed nor wanted such a change. In this particular hearing, objectors were treated with irritation bordering on contempt. Several objectors concluded that the system appeared to be working as though it was based on a malevolent collusion between licensees and licensing authorities. Reports suggested that this sequence of events was repeated all over England and Wales. The Government had given assurances that the new licensing arrangements would give more say to local communities over licensing matters. Events on the ground indicated otherwise. In fact, the wishes of local community members were being flagrantly ignored. Many objectors were informed that, even though they were being affected by nuisance from intoxicated or rowdy drinkers from a local pub, they could not give evidence unless they lived within 100 metres of it. In September 2005 the Government admitted that local authorities and the police had to operate under guidelines that were biased in favour of licensees wishing to open for longer hours. Within days of the new opening hours taking effect it was reported that:

> 'Thousands of rowdy pubs and clubs have been granted permission to open until the early hours because licensing boards are powerless to object... Despite repeated claims by Tessa Jowell, the Culture Secretary, that the Licensing Act gives new powers to local communities, the boards are powerless to reject complaints when 'interested parties', such as the police or environmental health officers, do not step in.' (Coates *et al.* 2005).

The suggestion, in September 2005, that the proposed new police powers to deal with 'persistent binge drinkers' and unruly bars provoked an angry response from some people, who warned of a new threat to civil rights. Ms Shami Chakrabati, Director of Liberty, reportedly commented on Tony Blair's proposals for the new police powers in these words:

'They are no longer investigating crime but dishing out punishments themselves. If he goes any further than he has already gone, he will be modifying policing in this country for all time.' (Travis 2005b).

'So 1984 is here. Not only will the police get the power to dispense summary justice, but drunken yobs are described as 'persistent binge drinkers'. Yet more Newspeak. I am a 'persistent binge drinker' in that I drink more than eight units in one session several times a week. It is the 'only on a special occasion' binge drinker who is more likely to get drunk. But even then, drink is an exacerbation to yobbishness, not an excuse for it.' (Downing 2005)

Practical problems

The proposed new licensing laws have been beset by a number of practical problems. Firstly, it emerged that to gain a new liquor licence involved completing a complex, legalistic, 26 page form that few people could understand. This discouraged many licensees from submitting their applications to renew (or alter) their licenses on time. Many failed to do this by the deadline of August 8th 2005.

Because of this, approximately 20,000 bars were reportedly given permission to operate illegally until the confusion was cleared up. As noted above, Alcohol Disorder Zones had been created by the Government in order to facilitate the reduction of alcohol-related crime and public nuisance. It was reported in June 2005 that thousands of licensed premises might be exempt from paying the charges to be imposed on licensees within these zones. This was because nightclubs could escape such payment because their owners could claim that selling alcoholic drinks was not their main activity (Whitehead 2005a).

Local councils

Under the new arrangements local councils are responsible for the granting of liquor licenses in England and Wales. One official charged with this new responsibility informed the authors that this was a 'logistical nightmare, with too much to do in too little time'. A report in the *Sunday Times* has claimed that some councils in areas that are 'blighted by binge drinking are refusing new licences to pubs, clubs and bars that want to open late'. (Ungoed-Thomas and Winnett 2005).

The debate about licensing arrangements fits into the bigger picture of the overall approach to alcohol policy of New Labour. Throughout the strident and continuing debate about these controversial plans, two things have been especially striking. The first is the reticence of the Department of Health. The latter has remained almost silent during this discussion, even though alcohol policy is a major health issue. Secondly, alcohol policy is supposed to be implemented by all relevant departments cooperating. This does not seem to have happened.

The recent fierce debate about licensing law has taken place against a background of strong and growing concern about the problems associated with 'binge drinking'. This was given impetus by a number of research findings. These included the announcement and publication in November and December 2004 of the results of the UK part, then the international findings of, the European School Survey Project on Alcohol & other Drugs (ESPAD) 2003 (M.A. Plant and M.L. Plant 2004, Hibell *et al.* 2004). These received widespread media coverage and comment. The intensity of the opposition to extended licensing hours has been remarkable. The diversity of the coalition voicing opposition to this development has also been striking. All-day drinking has emerged as having few real supporters. In view of this, the Government has reacted by distancing itself from this particular proposal while attempting to sanitize the intended legal changes by attempts to moderate some of the possible harmful effects.

Chapter 6

Lessons from the past

Prior to the 2001 election in the United Kingdom, the Labour Party sent out a text message to young voters stating: 'cdnt give a XXXX 4 lst ordrs? Vote labour on thrsdy 4 xtra time'. (BBC News Online 2004c). The 2003 Licensing Act for England and Wales fulfils this implied promise: in contrast to previous legislation, it 'does not prescribe the days or the opening hours when alcohol may be sold by retail for consumption...' (Department of Culture, Media & Sport 2005). The premise which underlies this statement is that this liberalisation of licensing laws will reduce the problems associated with heavy or inappropriate drinking.

The UK Government has embarked upon a policy of liberalising public bar opening hours in the face of widespread opposition. The theory behind this move is that harmful drinking practices are the result of drinking against the clock just before bar closing time. It is suggested that the limited bar opening hours foster heavy drinking in the time available and the continuing rise in alcohol-related assaults and associated bad behaviour (Travis 2005c p.10).

Some Government ministers have suggested that the removal of the 'six o'clock swill' will encourage the British to adopt a relaxed, continental style of drinking. The Licensing Minister Richard Caborn has suggested that the proposed changes will bring an end to binge drinkers dominating streets (BBC News Online 2005d). A Home Office representative has stated: 'Indeed in many countries that have more liberalised licensing hours, binge drinking is far less frequent' (BBC News Online 2005c,d). In fact the Government has not produced any peer-reviewed scientific evidence that supports their claims (E. J. Plant and M. A. Plant 2005).

The new flexibility of permitted hours for licensed premises is intended to be applied subject to '...the expert opinion of a range of authorities in relation to the licensing objectives'. Four licensing objectives are listed: The prevention of crime and disorder, public safety, the prevention of public nuisance and the protection of children from harm. The objectives, unlike their Scottish counterparts, do not include a reference to protecting public health.

Is binge drinking really the 'unintended' consequence of restricted licensing hours as Culture Secretary Tessa Jowell, whose Department of Culture, Media and Sport (DCMS) is supervising the licensing amendments, would have people believe? (BBC News Online 2002a). It is true that the British now expect much more flexible options for shopping and entertainment. Entertainment, is of course, central to the DCMS plans for the act: entertainment and liquor licences will be combined, dramatically reducing costs to the licensee (BBC News Online 2002c). The expectation being that a more musical, cultural nightlife will develop in addition to expected tourism benefits. The problem is that the British already have a long established drinking culture. As outlined in Chapter 1, this has long been noted to feature heavy drinking, especially during weekend evenings. Alcohol is clearly not the same as most other consumer goods; its effects on health and behaviour should lead to the adoption of evidence-based policies to reduce such adverse effects (Smith 1988).

Professor Ian Gilmore, Chairman of the Royal College of Physicians College's Licensing Committee, has dubbed the suggestion that the British will adopt a more continental style of consumption in light of the liberalisation as 'fanciful' (BBC News Online 2005f). The College predicts instead an increase in alcohol-related problems which could cost the UK's National Health Service millions of pounds (The Telegraph Online 2005). Furthermore the College warns that the act could change the nature of Britain's drinking problem (BBC News Online 2004c). Even should it effectively reduce alcohol-related disorder the act may very well also prolong the period when it occurs; with all emergency services having to redeploy resources accordingly. International evidence which supports this claim will be examined shortly.

The outgoing London Metropolitan Police Commissioner, Sir John Stevens, has voiced similar concerns from a public order perspective, emphasising that resources will have to be reassigned away from other duties to cover the period of extended opening (BBC News Online 2005f). In addition, unpublished Home Office research indicates a link between binge drinking and a 14% increase in violent crime, a significant proportion of which occurs near licensed premises, with 47% of victims believing their assailant was under the influence of alcohol (Lewis, in Leppard and Winnett 2005). The potential for increasing police time being devoted to alcohol-fuelled antisocial behaviour is real and the possible impact on both morale and recruitment must also be considered.

In addition to an extended period when police will have to deal with the fallout of excessive drinking, further duties will be placed upon their shoulders under the provisions of the new act. The introduction of safeguards such as 48 hour shut-downs for premises selling to minors and on-the-spot fines for irresponsible alcohol service will add to policing work (BBC News Online 2005e,g). The police already have at their disposal exclusion and anti-social behaviour orders to ban problem drinkers from pubs and town centres and on-the spot fines for those causing a nuisance on the streets (Turner 2004). These powers are rarely employed. In view of this it must be asked whether adding to an infrequently deployed arsenal will really help.

As outlined earlier, the widely criticised *Alcohol Harm Reduction Strategy for England* is an emasculated version of a more credible interim evidence review (M.A. Plant 2004a). The draft report included some of the findings from international studies on the adverse effects of extending licensing hours to be discussed shortly. This evidence did not appear in the finished strategy report prompting accusations that the document had been effectively 'sexed-down' (BBC News Online 2004c).

It has been suggested that Culture Secretary Tessa Jowell, a strong supporter of licensing liberalisation, may have been influenced by the advice of The Portman Group, a beverage alcohol industry organisation (Robbins 2005). That the influence of industry is weighty indeed is not surprising. This influence appears to be at least a factor in the Government's unwilling-ness to acknowledge the effectiveness of stricter control options such as taxation and its emphasis on largely ineffective strategies like education. This influence appears to be so strong that Room has characterised it as a 'veto' (in BBC News Online 2005c). Such measures as taxation, politically unpopular in an election year, are also financially distasteful for the alcohol industry. There was originally a suggestion that the industry would be expected to contribute to the extra cost of policing the new bar opening hours. This was vetoed. Even so, this policy has since been partly reversed (in the form of increased costs for bar owners) as part of a package of measures announced by the Government in January 2005 in the face of widespread hostility to the planned new arrangements (E. J. Plant and M. A. Plant 2005).

There has been remarkable unanimity among scientific and medical author-ities in the UK that the proposed liberalisation is ill-conceived. Furthermore such liberalisation is not 'a leap in the dark' as former Home Secretary David Blunkett has claimed (Leppard and Winnett 2005). Studies regarding the effects of extended opening hours have been conducted in several countries. This information will now be examined.

Lessons from the past

British experience

Restrictions on the licensing of the sale of alcohol were introduced by Edward VI in 1552. Since then a degree of control has been part of the British scene. As outlined in Chapter 1, all-day licensing has been tried before in the form of the 1830 Beer Act. This increased both alcohol consumption and alcohol problems.

Some international experiences

Availability theory holds that increasing the availability of alcohol will lead to increased consumption and, consequently, increased harm (Ragnarsdottír et al. 2002 p.146). The evidence indicates that, more often than not, it does.

Iceland

In 1999 Reykjavik Municipal Council experimented with liberalised opening hours for bars and restaurants. In Iceland, as subsequently in the UK, proponents of liberalisation predicted it would spread police workload more evenly and reduce problem drinking. Ragnarsdottír et al. (2005) concluded that there were indeed positive results regarding workload for both the police nightshift and the hospital accident and emergency department (A&E), neither of which experienced the same post-closing peaks as they had before. Taxi-queues were also found to have shortened.

The total numbers of admissions to the A&E were, however, found to have increased after controls were relaxed. Drink-driving was estimated to have risen a remarkable 80% (Kjartansdottír, in BBC News Online 2005h). Local residents were also disturbed by the prolonged nightlife (Olafsdottír 2003). A police commander has speculated that increased drug dealing found in those bars with extended hours of operation may be the result of stimulants such as cocaine and amphetamines being taken to stay awake (Olafsdottír 2003a). Tourism costs were also high: with the nightlife stretching over into morning difficulties were encountered by those cleaning the streets, the appearance of the Reykjavik city centre suffering as a result. This was due in part to intoxicated people still leaving bars and clubs when families were venturing out the next day. Significantly, in 2001, the city council reinstituted restrictions on serving-hours at the request of the police and the City Centre Steering Group in response to growing alcohol-related problems around the city centre. (Ragnarsdottír et al. 2005). Olafsdottír (2005) has recently summarised Iceland's response to the adverse effects of extended hours as follows:

> 'What has happened in Reykjavík is that the regulations of opening hours have been clarified. Pubs in the city centre and in demarcated areas can apply for extended

opening hours on Friday and Saturday nights and the night before a public holiday. On the weekdays they are open to one o'clock. They can open again two hours later but are not allowed to sell alcoholic beverages until 11 o'clock. Neighbourhood restaurants, bars or pubs would not get permission for extended opening hours.'

Australia and Canada

Chikritzhs and Stockwell (2002) examined the impact of extended trading hours in Western Australia on the level of violent assault occurring in the vicinity of the public houses (termed 'hotels' in Australia) with later opening. Legislative changes since the early eighties have resulted in the liberalisation of licensing laws throughout Australia, a country whose drinking-style inspired the term the 'six o'clock swill' noted above. Australia has a drinking culture that is similar in many ways to that of the UK. Comparing pubs with Extended Trading Permits (ETPs) and pubs without, all of which had experienced similar monthly assault rates prior to the extensions being granted, the authors found there was a significant increase in assaults in or near pubs with ETPs. It was not shown whether the observed increase in alcohol sales in pubs with ETPs was due to increased patronage or increases in individuals' consumption although the authors surmised that both may have occurred. Significantly, trading hours in Perth were typically extended for only one hour at weekends and yet a 70% mean increase in violent assault resulted.

In both Australia and Canada studies have specifically examined the road safety impact of extended opening hours in public houses. In assessing the introduction of flexible trading hours in Tasmania, Smith (1988) found that, while premises tended to open for the same *total* number of hours, they generally opened later. This resulted in increased patronage and, consequently: increased consumption leading to a 'significant 10.8% increase in casualty traffic accidents' in comparison to the control period.

Vingilis *et al.* (2005) examined the impact of the 1996 extension of trading hours in Ontario from 1 to 2 a.m. The authors observed little change in the number of blood-alcohol positive road fatalities with the extension of trading hours. Vingilis *et al.* however highlight the minimal uptake for the extended opening among licensed establishments indicating that availability may not have increased much in real terms.

Ireland

In any case UK policy makers need not even look so far afield to study the results of liberalising licensing hours. Indeed, the problematic issue of the extension of licensing hours has already been encountered in England itself. In 1921, a Dr Shadwell noted a link between rising convictions for drunkenness and the liberalisation of trading hours in his book *Drink in 1914–1922: A Lesson in Control* (Shadwell in Commission on Liquor Licensing 2003).

Some of the most compelling evidence against extending the hours of alcohol sale comes from Ireland. The Intoxicating Liquor Act (2000) introduced later opening hours in the Republic of Ireland. Rationalisations similar to those currently being employed in the UK were behind the move such as restricted hours encouraging unsafe drinking patterns, accusations of paternalism; inconvenience for those working irregular hours and anticipated tourism benefits from bringing Ireland into line with much of Europe.

Irish pubs were allowed to open until 11 p.m. on Sundays; 11.30 p.m. Monday–Wednesday; and 12.30 a.m. Thursday–Saturday; plus thirty minutes 'drinking-up' time (Dáil Éireann 2000). Furthermore, clubs were allowed special exemptions until 2.30 a.m., also with a thirty minute drinking-up period. A number of negative consequences followed the introduction of these changes: binge-drinking, especially among under-age drinkers spiralled upwards (Kettle 2003). An increase in A&E attendances, between a quarter and a third of which are alcohol-related, was also observed (The Telegraph Online 2005). The Commission on Liquor Licensing, assessing the impact of the 2000 Act, noted a perceived increase in disorder, drunkenness, vandalism, and injury after the extension of trading hours among the public (Commission on Liquor Licensing 2003). The Gardaí (police) reported a significant increase in alcohol-related and public order offences between 2000 and 2001 with a concomitant strain on their resources. The number of alcohol-related offences rose from 12.4% to 17% overall of offences involving juveniles in the same period. Interestingly, publicans reported to the Commission that the economic benefits of longer opening hours were negated by the attendant costs. In addition, club-operators reported that the decreased margin of time between pub-closing and club-closing reduced the incentive for people to visit clubs and was damaging profit. The public health benefits of this were also mentioned. People in nightclubs may divide time between drinking and dancing, whereas those who only frequent pubs are more likely to drink throughout. Finally, strong anecdotal evidence was cited by the Commission of an increase in Friday absenteeism with the extension of Thursday night opening hours; resulting in a negative impact on work, training, and education.

During 2003 the Irish Government introduced a new Intoxicating Liquor Act to combat problems created by the act of 2000 (Butler 2003). A key measure of the new bill, in accordance with the recommendations of the Commission on Liquor Licensing, was the amendment of Thursday night closing time back to the original 11.30 p.m.

Scotland

Scotland is also facing the prospect of licensing changes (Johnston 2005). The Scottish Executive's 2004 white paper produced in response to a licensing law consultation document the Nicholson Report, states that there is a 'presumption against 24-hour opening in Scotland'. Scotland has already some experience of the extension of licensing hours. Foster (2003) observes that in 1976 limited deregulation occurred without a dramatic increase in alcohol problems. The author however cautions that Scotland was in the grip of a severe recession in 1976 and, as there is a clear link between alcohol consumption and disposable income, little can be drawn from these findings about the initial impact of the Scottish changes. Moreover, it has become evident in the past decade that Scottish rates of alcohol-related liver disease and alcohol dependence have increased substantially (M. A. Plant 2004b). The Nicholson Report itself noted the fivefold increase of acute alcohol-related hospital admissions in Scotland between 1980 and 2000 (Scottish Executive 2003).

The Office of Population Censuses and Survey (OPCS) reported in 1986 that consumption in Scotland had actually risen by 13% since the 1976 act came into force (Baggott 1990). This was largely due to an increase in female consumption and the report fell short of attributing this to the reforms in the licensing law. The OPCS report did not, however, examine the impact of the Scottish changes upon indicators of alcohol abuse such as the incidence of liver cirrhosis or drunk-driving. The results of those few studies which did attempt such analysis were inconclusive. Baggott attributes this to the complexity of the relationship between licensing laws, consumption and harm as being subject to many and varying interpretations.

Uptake

The issue of who would make use of extended hours is central to predicting their effect. In Australia the uptake of extended licensing was not high. A Licensing Commission survey performed after the introduction of flexible trading hours in Tasmania reported that most hotels opened for the same *number* of hours as before the changes: they simply opened later (Smith 1988, p.219). It must be noted however, that while the economic benefits from extended opening to small neighbourhood public houses may be prohibitive, to the large town centre 'superpubs' it may prove more financially viable. The outcome, should this prove an accurate assertion, remains to be seen. It was reported at one stage that the great majority (130,000) of licensed premises in England and Wales were granted extended opening hours before the advent of the new licensing arrangements. Over 700 of these licensed premises had been granted 24-hour licences (Whitehead 2005b). Later evidence from a subsequent BBC survey (noted above) suggested that about a third of pubs, clubs, and shops licensed to sell alcohol had been granted extended licences by November 23rd 2005. The same survey noted that only 359 pubs and clubs would be getting 24-hour licences. (BBC News Online 2005h).

There are several further considerations arising from the extent of longer opening hours. Foremost among these is that minimal changes in availability are unlikely to affect the predicted metamorphosis of Britain's 'inContinental drinkers' (Garretsen 2003) into wine-sipping continental-style consumers. Secondly, if the owners of many premises only request short licensing extensions, the public order and other problems associated with closing time may not be substantially changed.

There is a final, significant issue of uptake and here we may refer again to international evidence. The majority of evaluations from Scandinavia have examined the effects of reducing hours of sale from off-licenses rather than pubs, clubs or restaurants. One finding has obvious relevance to the changes outlined in the Licensing Act 2003. Mäkelä et al. (2002) conducted an in-depth literature review of documented alcohol control policies in Norway, Finland, and Sweden. It was found that reducing hours of alcohol sale, whether as deliberate government policy or through the 'natural experiment' of strikes, had the most significant effect on heavy drinkers' consumption, which decreased.

Accordingly Mäkelä et al. (2002) suggest that liberalisation is likely to have the greatest effect on those most restricted by the previous policy. In the case of the 2003 Licensing Act this may mean either those who wish to drink at different periods or those who wish to drink for longer periods. Room et al. (2002) offer some indication of just who will avail themselves of extended trading hours. Their study concluded that the majority of Nordic attempts at alcohol control, even those with no impact on overall consumption, had most effect on 'troublesome or social marginal drinkers' (Room et al. 2002 p.171).

Based upon the Nordic experience, it can be inferred that while moderate drinkers, such as those who would enjoy a glass of wine when they leave the theatre, may only be slightly affected by liberalised opening hours. In contrast, heavier (binge) drinkers may be much more affected. It surely must follow that it is not moderate drinkers who would take advantage of extended drinking hours, but rather those who have already demonstrated themselves lacking in the type of restraint the Government seems to be hoping for. Evidence from the 1987 America's Cup supports this theory; those with extant high levels of consumption were found most likely to capitalise upon the liberalisation of serving-hours (McLaughlin, in Chikritzhs and Stockwell 2002 p.592).

The UK Government appears therefore to be relying on people to not begin drinking earlier or even at the same time as they did prior to liberalisation. It also appears to be relying on them not drinking more than they currently do. International evidence clearly does not support this expectation. It does however offer some alternatives. Smith (1988) suggests that, since one reason given by the leisure industry for wanting flexible trading hours is that they could close during uneconomically quiet periods, allowing flexible opening within set opening and closing times would be a good compromise. In both Tasmania and Iceland the concept of 'drinking-up time' has been developed with good results. While remaining open later, premises stop serving alcohol and providing entertainment a whole hour before closing, thereby alleviating the pressure to rush the last drink or to leave the premises in a crowd.

Whether legislation should lead or follow popular opinion is a complex issue. It may be unrealistic to expect that draconian restrictions on alcohol sale will be introduced by the industry-friendly UK Government. The current UK Government appears to be anxious to avoid accusations of 'nannying'; despite the fact that the scope and severity of the problem indicate that 'a bit of nannying is quite in order' (Drummond in Johnston 2005). The rate of alcohol-related mortality in the UK is rising steadily and some form of effective action clearly needs be taken. It should, however, be acknowledged that a stronger case can be made for taking no action than following the Government's current course of increasing the availability of a substance that is already causing massive problems related to health and disorder.

Binge-drinking was less of a problem when deregulation of licensing hours was first proposed in the late 1990s. Now, however, it has effectively overtaken the legislation. In forming this legislation the Government had access to the information contained in this Chapter. Past experience suggests that the new licensing arrangements risk leading to a rise in heavy drinking, illicit drug use, violence, morbidity, and traffic accidents. The lack of attention the UK Government has apparently devoted to the experience of other countries where on sale availability has been extended is remarkable. The UK has a serious 'alcohol problem'. This really requires a far more coherent and consistent response designed to alleviate the associated health and social problems. Alcohol-related problems are fostered by many social, psychological, and other factors, not the least of which is the UK's longstanding traditional patterns of drinking. It is acknowledged that greatly reducing such problems is a big challenge. Even so, it does appear to be very unwise to introduce a policy that has a considerable prospect of aggravating the current position.

Chapter 7

Future directions?

'It is undeniable that a gigantic evil remains to be remedied, and hardly any sacrifice would be too great which would result in a marked diminution of this national degradation.'
(Report of the Royal Commission on Liquor Licensing Laws, 1896–1869, cited by Wilson (1940 p.259))

'Prevention is not just printing leaflets.' (Gmel 2005)

'How to minimise the harm of alcohol in ways that are politically and socially viable should be the goal so that the swings from one extreme to the other are smoothed out and health and safety improve.' (Musto 1997)

'Reducing the harm that can be done by alcohol is one of the greatest public health challenges facing the European Region of WHO. Ways of talking up this challenge are well known. What is needed now is to exercise political will, to mobilise civil society and carry out systematic programmes in every member State.' (World Health Organization 1994)

Just imagine .... a gas begins to seep out of the ground beneath our feet. Not all the time, mainly during the evenings. Millions of people inhale this gas. It has an effect on them. Some drive their cars into walls and die, often killing and injuring others in the process. Some attack other people. Some commit rape. In many areas citizens are afraid to venture out after dark because of their fear of the prowling gas-afflicted predators. Some people suffer serious organ damage and die from cancers or other diseases. Some women give birth to seriously damaged children. These grow up to be permanently damaged and disabled both mentally and physically. Some people become addicted to inhaling the gas and lose their ability to live happy, fulfilling lives.

What should the Government do about this crisis? Should it:

- Print warning notices and fund health education campaigns
- Arm the police
- Issue gas masks
- Recruit more undertakers
- Fence off the gas vents
- Bomb the gas vent areas

- Call in Bruce Willis

OR

- SHOULD IT TURN OFF THE GAS? (OR AT LEAST, TURN IT DOWN?)

Many people would probably support the last option.

Is alcohol different from toxic gas? Yes and no. Firstly, the effects of alcohol are related to what people choose to drink and the pattern and level of consumption. One drink probably won't hurt you, but several might do so. A lot will do. Large quantities of alcohol can be poisonous. Secondly, moderate alcohol consumption is popular, enjoyable, and legal. As noted earlier in this book, moderate consumption does have some health benefits, at least for the middle aged and elderly. Conversely, it is evident that the harm associated with alcohol consumption can be reduced by public policy if this substantially reduces heavy drinking.

There are two rather different traditions in relation to how to deal with the problems associated with alcohol. One of these is known as the 'Public Health approach'. The other is known as 'Harm minimisation' or 'Harm reduction'.

The Public Health approach sets out to reduce the level of alcohol-related problems by reducing the overall level of alcohol consumption. This is justified by the fact that, in general, the level of alcohol problems in a society rises and falls in association with trends in alcohol consumption. There is a lot of evidence to support this perspective. This approach is supported by some of the leading alcohol researchers (Bruun *et al.* 1975, Edwards *et al.* 1995, Babor *et al.* 2003). It has, however, been criticised as being akin to 'draining the ocean to prevent shark attacks' (Rehm 1999).

Harm minimisation is designed to reduce the level of problems associated with alcohol without necessarily reducing overall alcohol consumption. The key considerations for successful harm minimisation measures have been identified as:

'Have they worked?
Are they transferable to other contexts?
Are they politically/socially acceptable?'
(M.A. Plant *et al.* 1997).

This approach really echoes the goals of some of the early British Temperance campaigners. The latter sought to foster moderate and harm-free drinking rather than aiming to introduce total prohibition.

Evidence of 'what works' is available and has been reviewed by several commentators (e.g. M.A. Plant *et al.* 1997, Babor *et al.* 2003, Stockwell *et al.* 2005). There is a high level of scientific agreement about most aspects of what the evidence has shown. Even so, researchers have differed in relation to some of their personal conclusions about which policies should be pursued most vigorously.

What are the policy options? The evidence in brief

Alcohol is important. Most adolescents and adults in Britain enjoy drinking it. Alcohol is not only widely used and a well-established part of our society, it is often in the news, if all too frequently because of the harm associated with heavy or inappropriate consumption. It is a remarkable fact that few people appear to be aware of what the scientific evidence really shows in relation to alcohol control policies and their impact. There is big gulf between the evidence and public and political awareness. This is exemplified by the periodic declarations by politicians such as Tessa Jowell that their administrations will respond to binge drinking and other related problems with expensive alcohol education or publicity campaigns. Such initiatives are politically attractive because they are a conspicuous way of demonstrating to the public that some form of action is being taken. Some politicians hope that this symbolises political awareness as well as serious concern. Policies of this type are widely accepted, are not intrusive and do not cause inconvenience to people. There appears to be a widespread assumption that approaches of this type might discourage heavy drinking or reduce its associated ill effects. What is the evidence? This chapter sets out to highlight some of the information that is available about 'what works'. The policy approaches that are briefly considered in the following pages include alcohol education and health promotion, labelling, enforcing the existing laws such as those on drink driving, local community action, creating safer bars, restricting the access of young people to alcohol, and the use of taxation to curb alcohol consumption.

Alcohol education and health promotion

In fact, evidence shows very clearly that at this point in time neither education nor public campaigning about alcohol make much difference to the way in which a society views or consumes alcohol. Alcohol education and health promotion related to alcohol have been reviewed in great detail elsewhere (e.g. Kalb 1975, Kinder et al. 1980, Schaps et al. 1981, Bandy and President 1983, Tobler 1986, Edwards et al. 1995, M.A. Plant 1997, Babor et al. 2003, Crombie et al. 2005). Most scientists have concluded that this is simply not an effective way of reducing heavy drinking or alcohol problems in a population. It appears that alcohol education, often directed at secondary school pupils, sometimes raises knowledge and modifies attitudes. This effect is usually ephemeral, dissipating after a few weeks. A recent review by Foxcroft *et al.* (2003) concluded that only a tiny number of credible educational programmes had actually reduced young people's drinking. Such programmes appear to be very rare (Midford and McBride 2004, McBride 2005, Poulin and Nicholson 2005). Some alcohol education programmes appear to have increased what young people drink and, smoke as well as their illicit drug use (e.g. Hawthorne *et al.* 1995). This is not wholly surprising since the usual intended effect of any type of education is to raise interest and involvement. In the case of alcohol, it is clear that the social and psychological factors that mainly influence young people are family and other social pressures, including the drinking habits of their peers and role models.

In summary, alcohol education and health promotion campaigns, though often politically appealing, have been shown, with some rare exceptions, to have little or no positive effects on either drinking habits or alcohol-related problems.

Labelling

Labels have been used to provide warnings about alcohol and to give information about the alcohol content of different beverages. As Greenfield (1997) has reported, warning labels have been made mandatory in India, Mexico, and the USA:

> 'Mandatory warning labels may be justified by officials and the public on a right-to-know basis: consumers of the product are offered accurate information on which to base their choices about its use.' (p.105)

Warning labels were made compulsory in the USA in 1989 by order of Congress. The warnings relate to the dangers of birth defects resulting from maternal drinking during pregnancy and the risks associated with driving under the influence of alcohol or operating machinery after drinking. Evaluation of the impact of the US warning labels indicates that in the short-term public support for warning labels increased. In contrast, popular support for twelve other alcohol control policies remained unchanged (Hilton and Kaskutas 1991, Kaskutas 1993). Evidence that the warning labels influenced behaviour is meagre. Even so, it was evident that heavier drinkers, as expected, were more aware of the messages than were lighter drinkers. The impact of the warning labels has been summarised by Greenfield thus:

> 'Although not conclusive evidence of an effect due to the warning labels' messages, these findings are at least consistent with the Congressional intent, by showing that the appropriate groups are being reminded of the harms, and that other personal characteristics including drinking variables accounted for, those more exposed to

the message appear more likely than others to be adopting harm-reduction strategies related to drinking and driving, and possibly, drinking less per occasion when pregnant and having more conversations about drinking and pregnancy.' (p.118)

It has periodically been suggested that the labelling of alcohol containers with statements of their alcohol content should be introduced in the UK. Even so, this has not become mandatory. Tesco introduced a kind of labelling in 1989. Even so, such informative labelling has been introduced in Australia (in terms of 'standard drinks'). Many people in Britain clearly do not know what units or 'standard drinks' are. Recent evidence confirms that many people are confused by government advice about what 'sensible drinking' really is (Hope 2005). As noted above, standard drinks vary in different countries. Evidence about the impact of such labels appears to be very scarce. In spite of this, labelling could be a useful means of supporting messages about high and low risk alcohol consumption levels (Stockwell and Single 1997).

Enforcing the existing law

The pub has been an important focus of leisure time and a source of entertainment, food and refreshment in Britain for centuries. As noted in Chapter 1, there have been attempts to regulate behaviour in bars for a very long time. The UK, like most other countries, has a number of laws that apply to alcohol consumption in bars that cause concern. These relate to issues such as serving alcohol to children, serving people who are intoxicated, alcohol-impaired driving, public nuisance, and aggressive or violent behaviour. The subject of alcohol-impaired or drunken driving is considered in a separate section below. As indicated earlier in this book, many of the public order and associated problems linked with alcohol occur in and around bars and clubs. The police, being in the 'front line', have taken a lead in attempting to moderate such problems and have recently been active in cities such as Cardiff, (the TASC project, see below) and Manchester, (the Manchester City Centre Safe Project).

A notable local experiment was carried out by the police in Torquay in the early 1980s. This attractive seaside town, like many similar places, had experienced problems with rowdy holiday makers, especially during the summer. Much of the trouble was focused in and around harbour-side bars. Local police visited these bars and explained that they would be vigilant in enforcing the law in relation to permitted opening hours, serving intoxicated patrons, and underage drinking. They offered to help deal with troublesome patrons, and reminded bar staff of what the law was in relation to the good bar management. This advice was followed up with frequent, regular visits to bars in the target area by uniformed officers. The policy was enforced for a year. During this experimental period there was a 20% fall in recorded offences in Torquay (Jeffs and Saunders 1983). Strangely this productive experiment was apparently widely ignored. Even so, the police in Sussex subsequently followed up the Torquay venture with a similar initiative of their own. They reported that this achieved a worthwhile reduction in alcohol-related crimes (Sussex Police 1987). Rydon and Stockwell (1997) have reviewed a number of other attempts to reduce disorder associated with bars:

'An attempt to replicate the Jeffs and Saunders study in Sydney by Burns *et al.* (1995) met with the finding that recorded assaults actually increased during the intervention phase using community policing methods. The researchers suggested that this finding may have been due to greater opportunity for police officers to observe assaults and take action in the experimental area. An analysis of hospital admissions for alcohol-related admissions for assault-related injuries showed a decrease during the intervention period...'(p.222)

Local community action

A number of initiatives have gone beyond the types of policing used in Torquay, Sussex and Sydney. The best known and documented of these has taken place in Surfers' Paradise, a resort on Australia's Gold Coast. This town, like Torquay, had suffered from serious disorder and violence associated with pubs and clubs. In the case of Surfers' Paradise, these were centred around a place called Cavill Mall. This had created a bad reputation for the area. It had been described as being 'sleazy'. The Surfers' Paradise Safety Action Project was an initiative in which licensing authorities, the local Council, police, taxi operators, security companies, bar owners, and managers were mobilised to form a coalition. This coalition set about reducing levels of alcohol-related aggression and violence. The project was managed by an interagency steering committee and a project officer was appointed to implement the initiative. A code of practice was drawn up for bars and clubs. The project extended to issues such as public safety and security and the enforcement of licensing regulations.

'In essence, the project aimed to achieve a commitment from licensees to self-regulation by shifting the broad context of the licensed venues from being alcohol oriented to being entertainment oriented, with emphasis on sound responsible hospitality practices. This shift was achieved in part through the administration of the Risk Assessment Policy Checklist. This checklist is a tool devised to assess, amongst other things, how well management deal with the provision of liquor and pricing, what responsible practices are being used; and how venues promote entertainment as well as liquor.' (Graham and Homel 1997 p.185).

The impact of this wide-ranging initiative was monitored. The resulting evidence indicated that this scheme led to improved bar management and a decline in binge drinking, intoxication, aggression and violence. Importantly, it was also evident that the scheme had not simply displaced such problems to other areas (Homel *et al.* 1994). Graham and Homel concluded that:

'The reductions in intoxication were in turn the result of major improvements in management and service practices, evidenced by the reduced use of gimmicks, lower use of drinks promotions and happy hours, and a reduction in the unsolicited topping up of patrons' drinks'. (pp.186–7).

A more recent assessment of both the Surfers' Paradise experiment and similar ventures in other parts of Australia has been provided by Haines and Graham (2005):

'Subsequent replications of the Surfers' Paradise model in regional Australian towns (Hauritz *et al.* 1998), quite different in nature to Surfers' Paradise, also demonstrated impressive reductions in violence (56% reduction in aggressive incidents, 75% reduction in total physical assaults). Despite the initial success in Surfers' Paradise, in subsequent years sustainability became an issue, and violence levels in Surfers' Paradise eventually reverted to previous norms (Hauritz *et al.* 1998). Nevertheless, the results of the project strongly suggest that modification of the various factors associated with the risk of violence in the licensed environment can lead to at least temporary reductions in violence.' (p.166).

Another community action scheme to reduce alcohol-related violence linked to licensed premises has been undertaken in Stockholm. This venture, the STAD project and its impact, have been summarised thus:

'In Sweden, the number of licensed premises has increased markedly over the past 15 years. The ten-year community alcohol prevention programme started in 1996 in the northern part of central Stockholm. Main intervention components included community mobilisation, training of servers in responsible beverage service, and stricter enforcement of existing alcohol laws ... The results showed a decrease in alcohol-related problems at licensed premises. The number of premises that refused alcohol service to intoxicated patrons changed from 5% in 1996, to 47% in 1999, to 59% in 1998, and 68% in 2001. Changes in alcohol service occurred both in the project and control area. During the project period assaults decreased significantly by 29% in the project area but increased slightly in the control area. Policy initiatives were implemented by the licensing authority and by the police equally in all of Stockholm. The multi-component programme seems to have successfully reduced problems related to alcohol consumption at licensed premises. The most likely explanation for this is a combination of RBS training, building of community networks and policy routines initiated by the project. The results ... support earlier findings that multi-component interventions targeting licensed premises at the community level have the potential to reduce alcohol-related problems.' (Wallin and Andréasson 2005 p. 207).

A police-led initiative, Tackling Alcohol-Related Street Crime (TASC), was set up in Cardiff in July 2000. This venture involved a 'focused dialogue between the police and members of the licensed trade'. TASC involved the following elements:

> 'Measures aimed at improving the quality and behaviour of door staff.
> Attempts to influence licensing policy and practice.
> Measures aimed at publicising the problem of alcohol-related violent crime.
> Targeted policing operations directed at crime and disorder 'hot spots'.
> A cognitive behavioural programme for repeat offenders.
> A training programme for bar staff ('Servewise').
> A programme of education about alcohol for school-aged children.
> Support for victims of alcohol-related assaults attending hospital.' (Maguire and Nettleton 2003 p.v)

This exercise resulted in the following mixed outcomes:

> 'A comparison of the first 12 months after the launch of the project with the previous 12 months indicated an overall decrease of four per cent in incidents involving alcohol-related assaults. This occurred despite a ten per cent increase in licensed premise capacity in central Cardiff. During the same period, incidents of violence against the person rose elsewhere in South Wales... Virtually all the rise in disorder was accounted for by one street in Cardiff, which had the densest concentration of pubs and clubs and several newly opened premises... Overall, the TASC project was most successful in terms of targeted work with individual premises.' (Maguire and Nettleton 2003 p.vi)

The TASC project illustrates both what can be gained by the careful monitoring and control of problem bars and clubs and the limitations of attempts to operate in the context of large and expanding concentrations of licensed premises. Many people might think that it was remarkable that the number of licensed premises in central Cardiff was allowed to increase during the first year of the study. This area has clearly had a lot of alcohol problems for a long time. TASC has been a brave attempt to swim against a strong tide of increasingly available and ever cheaper alcohol served, in an expanding concentration of bars and clubs that mainly attract young people. In such areas there is clearly an ethos of heavy weekend drinking and aggression. One Cardiff resident informed the authors that: 'This area is notorious. People just avoid it unless they want to get drunk.'

It would be reasonable to conclude that TASC might have been far more productive if not inhibited both by local licensing policy and the national trends of cheaper and more readily available alcohol. Local licensing policy appears to have been working in a way that had probably damaged the prospects of TASC achieving major positive results. As noted elsewhere in this book, it is evident that licenses have been granted in urban areas where neither public safety nor public health justify them.

Creating safer bars

The impact of large concentrations of licensed premises and the size of bars on heavy drinking, intoxication, and disorder has been considered in Chapter 3. There is a lot of additional evidence demonstrating that there is a connection between the nature of a bar (its appearance, amenities, and management) and the levels of heavy drinking and aggression that occur in and near it (Graham 1985, Graham and Homel 1997). A pioneering study of Vancouver bars indicated that aggression was linked to bars that were grubby, poorly maintained, and with unattractive décor (Graham *et al.* 1980). The researchers reported that poor physical bar environment gives patrons their first cue about what type of behaviour might be tolerated. They also concluded that the following factors were associated with aggressive barroom behaviour:

'Overall decorum expectations (rated from 'restrictive' to 'anything goes'), swearing, (especially abusive swearing), sexual activity among patrons, sexual competition, prostitution, drug use and dealing, male rowdiness and male roughness or bumping.' (p.177)

Homel (*et al.* 1994) also concluded from Australian research that poor bar hygiene was associated with aggression. Graham and Homel have noted that aggression in bars is associated with poor ventilation and smoky air, poor access to the bar, high noise levels and crowding. These have commented:

'Because these relationships were identified in observational studies, it is not known whether these factors actually caused or contributed to aggression in some way, whether these attributes are simply more common in bars where aggression occurs due to other causes. However, it is known from the experimental literature on alcohol and aggression that drinking increases the likelihood of aggression in situations where there is frustration or provocation. Therefore, a plausible link between these aspects of the environment and aggressive behaviour is the role of these factors in irritating, frustrating or otherwise provoking bar patrons, particularly intoxicated bar patrons.' (p.174)

Some bars attract a lot of people who are 'high risk' in relation to heavy drinking. As explained in Chapter 2 of this book, such consumption is particularly commonplace among those in their late teenage years and in their early twenties. The traditional assumption has been that males were the problem group here. Recent social changes now mean that young women often drink heavily and get involved in disorder and aggression. It has been shown that the identified risk factors in bars include groups of males who are strangers, the presence of underage girls, drunken people with money to spend, and an 'anything goes' atmosphere (Homel *et al.* 1992, 1994, Fagan 1993).

Music has been shown sometimes to be a factor in heavy drinking or aggression. A study by Bach and Shaefer (1979) indicated that the speed of drinking was inversely related to the tempo of country music being played in a bar! Slow music was associated with fast drinking and vice versa. Homel *et al.* (1992) concluded that although noise was a factor in aggression, loud music in bars did not necessarily have bad effects. They found that a good live band would capture people's attention while a bad one provoked boredom and aggression.

Graham and Homel have concluded generally that the least attractive bars tend to be frequented by the most aggressive people. They recommended banning chronic trouble makers and training bar staff. There is evidence to suggest that most of those who frequent bars support the introduction and operation of some policies to keep them safe and orderly (e.g. Ratcliffe and Nutter 1979). One of the main reasons for training bar staff is to enable them to 'cut-off' or handle intoxicated or ill-behaved drinkers in the most efficient and diplomatic manner. Server training is mainly intended to ensure that bar staff do not serve people who are drunk and/or badly behaved. The problem is that high blood alcohol levels are associated with aggression, but they are also associated with the level of bar profits. Responsible bar management means that running a peaceful bar should be as important a requirement for running a successful and profitable business. Saltz (1997), reviewing the literature in this field, noted that:

> 'More generally the rubric of Responsible Beverage Service (RBS) . . . refers to the steps that servers of alcoholic beverages can take to reduce the chances of their patrons (or guests) becoming intoxicated in the first place.' (p.72)

It is important that bar staff should reduce aggression, not provoke it. Bar staff vary considerably in their ability to curb aggression (Waring and Sperr 1982). There has been some evidence that door attendants or 'bouncers' have sometimes been the cause of aggression in the past (e.g. Homel *et al.* 1992).

Graham (1985) has described a number of government regulated changes that were introduced in bars in Alberta, Canada:

> 'These changes included: partitioning of large beer halls, improvements in décor, reduced size of bar, and dress codes. Apparently these changes were instituted in response to unruly behaviour and, although there seems to have been no scientific evaluation of these changes . . . persons interviewed at the time (such as bar managers, Liquor Control Board Officials) perceived the changes as extremely successful in improving behavior of bar patrons.' (Zarun 1978 p.73)

There is evidence that the use of toughened or safety glasses in bars is helpful in reducing accidental and non-accidental glass injuries (Shepherd 1994, Shepherd and Brinkley 1996, M.A. Plant *et al.* 1994). Safety glasses generally do not shatter into dagger-like shards when broken, unlike regular glass. They crumble into fragments rather like car windscreens. They are also more durable than non-safety glass. Glasses are often used as weapons in bar fights and have inflicted many serious and disfiguring facial injuries. The value of safety glass has been extended in the town of Taunton, England, where shops in the town centre have been fitted with this type of glass in their windows.

It is evident that a number of measures can reduce problems associated with licensed premises. It has been stressed by Donnelly and Briscoe (2005) that the most effective interventions should ideally be devised on the basis of evidence of what the problems really are.

Drink drive laws

Alcohol consumption seriously impairs a driver's ability to react quickly in event of an emergency. It also reduces a driver's chances of driving safely. One area where there has been success in many industrial countries, including the UK, is that of alcohol-impaired or drunken driving. This was once a much bigger problem that it has been recently, as shown in Figs. 3.11 and 3.12 in chapter 3 (Transportation Research Board 1994, Stewart and Sweedler 1997). In fact alcohol-impaired driving and related deaths have decreased in a number of countries with rather different legal approaches to this problem. There is no doubt that introduction of the breathalyser in the UK in 1967 combined with growing public disapproval of drunken driving have saved a lot of lives. This provided a crucial objective means of applying the law in this area. There is scope for further gains in this area since it is evident that reducing the Blood Alcohol Concentration (BAC) limit has saved lives in places such as Australia and the USA. It should be noted that such reductions have been strongly opposed by the beverage alcohol industry (Moore 1992, Stewart and Sweedler 1997). The BAC limit in the UK is currently 0.08% while in countries such as France and the Netherlands it is lower, 0.05%. Sweden has a legal BAC limit of 0.02%. In addition, it is evident that both random breath testing and rigorous enforcement of drink drive laws can be effective in reducing both the incidence of drink driving and related accidents (Homel *et al.* 1988, Moloney 1995, Henstridge *et al.* 1997, Stewart and Sweedler 1997). However, information must be provided on how much alcohol it takes to reach the legal blood alcohol limit. Breathalysers in bars are of some use. Even so, if someone has been drinking a lot of alcohol in a relatively short space of time, their blood alcohol level will continue to rise for some time after leaving the bar.

The advent of 'zero tolerance' laws for drink driving in the USA in some states in 1995 also led to substantial falls in alcohol-related driver accidents among both older and younger drivers (Hingson *et al.* 1997). The incidence of this type of accident amongst younger drivers was reduced in the USA by raising the minimum drinking age. This is discussed in the following section.

Restricting the access of young people to alcohol

'...one thing we do know for sure is that raising the minimum drinking age to 21 in the United States has saved many thousands of lives.' (Bonnie 2003 p.xvi)

The minimum age at which alcohol consumption is permitted in the UK is not 18 years as widely supposed, but 5 years. Even so, it is only permissible for people to buy alcohol and to consume it in bars if they are aged 18 years or older. The only 'official' reference to changing this position within Britain was the Erroll Committee's suggestion in 1972 that the age should be reduced to 16 years. Some countries have no minimum drinking age and in others it is as high as 20 or 21. Many have opted for a minimum age of 18 years. In fact, there is compelling evidence from the USA that raising the minimum legal drinking and alcohol purchase age does reduce youthful drinking and alcohol-related traffic accidents, injuries and fatalities (e.g. Klepp *et al.* 1996, O'Malley and Wagenaar 1981, Saffer and Grossman 1987, Wagenaar and Maybee 1986, Voas *et al.* 1999), (cited by Bonnie and O'Connel 2003).

It is evident that selling and serving alcohol to minors is a major problem in Britain. A nationwide police exercise during 2004 involved 'sting operations' in 1,825 licensed premises. This detected the illegal sale of alcohol to children in 650 of these establishments. Altogether 51% of the on-licences (bars) and 32% of the off-licences examined were selling to underage individuals (Manchester Online 2004).

Policies are not necessarily transferable from one country to another. Nations differ in their cultures, traditions, and forms of myopia. An eminent alcohol researcher from the USA recently asked one of the authors why the British, faced with an epidemic of binge drinking, did not tackle the problem by raising the legal drinking age. The reply he received was: 'We'll probably do this when Americans ban guns'.

Taxation

Next to prohibition, taxation is by far the most controversial method for controlling the level of alcohol consumption and its associated problems. In a society such as Britain in which most people drink, prohibition is not even on the outer margins of the policy agenda. Can the same be said of taxation? The politics of this contentious issue are considered later in this chapter.

It is clear that alcohol, like other commodities, is responsive to price. It has been shown in Fig. 2.8 (Chapter 2) that as the affordabilty of alcohol (as a proportion of family expenditure) has increased, so the level of consumption has risen. Alcohol taxation has been an important source of government revenue in the UK for a long time. It has been used to pay for wars and a host of other national activities. It has even periodically been used to curb alcohol consumption at times when the latter was identified as being a sufficiently big problem. Under most circumstances, however, alcohol taxes have been gauged to raise income without killing the goose that lays the golden egg. Government decisions about alcohol taxation have clearly been influenced by pressure from the beverage alcohol industry. As described previously, there has been a considerable increase in per capita alcohol consumption in the UK during recent decades. This is certainly the main reason why some alcohol-related problems have increased. Tobacco has been taxed as an important UK health measure since November 1995 (Hansard 1995). Alcohol has not been targeted in this way in spite of the extensive health, economic and social harm associated with heavy drinking.

Godfrey (1997) has described the position of alcohol taxation in these terms:

'Governments have a long tradition of taxing the goods people want to buy to raise revenue. Alcoholic beverages have, in most countries, borne a higher rate of tax than the average. However, home produced beverages are often favoured with lower rates of tax compared to those which are mainly imported. The setting of tax levels is subject to a number of pressures including the campaigning of the beverage alcohol industry. Decisions about the comparative levels and structures across different beverages may, as a result of these pressures, seem haphazard.' (p.29)

Taxation works by manipulating the price of alcohol. If it is to be employed as a public health measure, price increases should lead people to drink less and alcohol problems should also fall. It is well-established that alcohol consumption is responsive to price changes. Price could be used to influence alcohol consumption levels (Leung and Phelps 1993, Österberg 1995, Godfrey 1997).

As Godfrey has reported, the responsiveness of alcohol to price changes depends upon the popularity of each particular type of drink. Popular drinks, such as beer, tend to be less responsive or 'price elastic' than less popular beverages. As wine has become more popular, it has become less responsive to price changes than it used to be when it was not so widely consumed (Godfrey 2004).

There is evidence that some drinkers may be especially responsive to price changes. Godfrey has cited a US study by Chaloupka and Weschler (1995). This indicated that binge drinkers were more responsive to price change than were other drinkers. Other US studies have suggested that price rises particularly influence alcohol consumption among young drinkers (e.g. Grossman *et al.* 1987, Coate and Grossman 1988, cited by Babor *et al.* 2003, p.110). Scandinavian experience shows that a price increase may have the biggest impact on the heaviest drinkers. Price changes have also influenced the levels of alcohol-related problems (Room 2002). A British study by Sutton and Godfrey (1995) of males aged 18–24 years also suggested that heavier drinkers are more responsive to price changes than lighter drinkers. It has also been suggested that alcohol consumption among young people is especially likely to be responsive to price changes (Cook and Moore 1993, Moore and Cook 1995, Grossman *et al.* 1988).

Some studies have concluded that moderate drinkers may be more affected by a price change than heavier drinkers (e.g. Manning *et al.* 1995). These authors appear to have revised their view to a degree (Farrell *et al.* 2003). As Godfrey has reported, there is also clear evidence that price increases have the effect of reducing the rates of alcohol problems. Several studies support this conclusion. These have charted falls in a number of problems in association with increased alcohol prices. These problems include liver cirrhosis deaths (Cook 1981, Cook and Tauchen 1982) and drink driving deaths (Chaloupka *et al.* 1991, Saffer and Grossman 1987).

The link between the price of alcohol and the levels of a number of alcohol-related problems have been succinctly summarized thus:

> 'Several studies have examined the impact of the price of alcoholic beverages on homicides and other crimes, including rape, robbery, assaults, motor vehicle thefts, domestic violence, and child abuse (Cook and Moore 1993; Sloan *et al.* 1994; Chalpoupka *et al.* 1998; Markowitz and Grossman 1998, 2000). These studies suggest that raising the price of alcohol is likely to result in a reduction of violence. What is most striking about these studies is their convergence upon a single theme: raising alcohol taxes will lead to a reduction in a host of undesirable outcomes related to alcohol use.' (Babor *et al.* 2003 p.112)

Australia has used tax to reduce the price of weaker beers (Hall 2005 a,b). This has reportedly reduced heavy drinking and alcohol problems (Stockwell 2004 a,b).

Godfrey has provided a useful summary of the potential role of taxation:

> 'There is considerable evidence for the positive effects of tax in reducing harms in the USA where tax is relatively low. There is a paucity of similar studies set

in other countries and such policy comparisons would vary across time and countries. However, the available research does suggest that price rises are likely to result in fewer problems and that tax changes should be considered alongside more direct problem-oriented approaches.' (pp.37–8)

She has also added that in the case of the UK: 'a 10% price increase would lead to a 10% fall in consumption—other things being equal'. (Godfrey 2005). Godfrey has also calculated that to reduce UK per capita alcohol consumption to its 1979 level a 16% rise in taxation would be required (Leigh *et al.* 2005).

Robin Room, an internationally acknowledged expert on alcohol policy has commented:

'The general point that heavier drinkers are more or less proportionately affected by taxes (which means that in terms of **amount** of alcohol their change is greater) is pretty well-established.' (Room pers. comm.)

Public opinion appears to be mainly supportive of the least effective types of alcohol control policy. Surveys of US public opinion concerning control options indicate that people there were most supportive of low–medium impact policies such as warning labels, health education, treatment, and responsible beverage service policies in bars. More effective policies such as higher alcohol taxes and more restrictive hours of sale had less support (Greenfield *et al.* 2004). Commenting on these findings, Greenfield and Giesbrecht (2005) have suggested that there is a need to raise public awareness of the potential impact of 'environmentally oriented alcohol policies and their public health benefits'. A similar recommendation had been made earlier by the Royal College of Psychiatrists (1986). The BBC's Healthy Britain Survey indicated that 38% of respondents supported raising the price of alcohol and 23% supported raising the minimum drinking age to 21 years. In addition, 51% supported banning drinks' promotions and 87% supported the allocation of extra public funds to enforce the minimum age of alcohol sales (BBC 2004). The National Organisation for Fetal Alcohol Syndrome-UK (NOFAS-UK) is a charity dedicated to reducing alcohol-related birth damage. This agency commissioned a YOUGOV survey to examine public opinion concerning the use of warning labels. The results of this study were released in November 2005. This revealed that 71% of those surveyed supported the introduction of US-style warning labels for drivers and those operating machinery. In addition, 67% supported the introduction of warning labels for pregnant women (National Organisation for Fetal Alcohol Syndrome-UK 2005).

It is clear that public opinion is flexible and can be influenced (e.g. Lemmens *at al.* 1999). This has recently been demonstrated by the considerable growth of opposition to extended liquor licensing hours in England and Wales noted in Chapter 5. The latter certainly reflects intensive critical media coverage. It should be emphasised that evidence strongly supports the use of taxation to increase and maintain the affordability of alcohol prices. This option was recently rejected by government minister Hazel Blears on the grounds that the alcohol industry is a big employer (Leigh, Evans and Gould 2005).

Working with the alcohol industry

'In the earlier days, when the population was scattered, when thousands of public houses and many private households brewed their own beer, when the publican was, in an arguable sense, 'mine host', and the public house was the principal social centre of the neighbourhood, the influence of the Trade as a corporate entity was comparatively small. The public house, regardless of party, at election times was at the disposal of any candidate who wished to bribe the electors. When however, the nation began to realise the necessity for legislative control and restriction of the sale of liquor in the public interest, the Trade, in turn, realised that necessity for combined effort in defence of its own interest, which has resulted in the creation of a political combination which, down at any rate, to the war, was probably the most powerful in the country.' (Wilson 1940. p.182.)

'Millions of people drink alcohol responsibly every day. No-one wants to stop that pleasure. But there is a growing problem on our town and city centre streets on Friday and Saturday nights. There are a lot of excellent partnership schemes up and down the country to tackle irresponsible drinking. I know the industry is working hard on codes of practice to ensure that we avoid advertising and manufacturing that glamorises binge drinking and attracts under age drinkers...
I want to give the industry a chance to build on the good work that I know is already out there and to prove that it is committed to tackling the problems of binge drinking.' (Tony Blair, Prime Minister Speaking at a seminar on Responsible Drinking, hosted by Diageo Great Britain, May 2004)

The evidence poses a moral challenge for society and not least for both government and the beverage alcohol industry. It is no longer justifiable to maintain that the best way (or even a tangible way) to reduce alcohol problems is through 'education'. The latter, should of course, not be abandoned completely. It is morally right to provide children and adults with information and sound advice. Sadly, in the case of alcohol, this usually has little effect on their behaviour. This is certainly bad news for politicians who may wish to avoid difficult decisions. It is also a bitter pill to swallow for representatives of sections of the beverage alcohol industry who are unenthusiastic about policies that would curb alcohol consumption and hit their profit margins.

The Portman Group, representing major sections of the UK alcohol industry, states on its website that it believes the following:

'An 'educate and prevent' approach is more effective than blanket controls. Alcohol harm reduction measures should target the minority who misuse alcohol rather than the responsible drinking majority.'

This should be taken as a statement of self-interest. It is certainly not a view that many objective reviewers of the scientific evidence would support. It should be emphasized that the alcohol industry is not monolithic. Some senior people in this industry do not share the Portman Group's views and have a genuine concern about the problems associated with their product. The industry as a whole should not be vilified because of the views and activities of only some of its representatives. Even so Government should keep any powerful industry firmly in check whenever it threatens public health and safety.

In view of alcohol education's poor track record, it is not credible to believe that it will lead to significant reductions in Britain's alcohol problems in the foreseeable future, if ever. To deny this is akin to the oil industry's reluctance to acknowledge that the burning of fossil fuels contributes to climate change and global warming. This stance threatens to put many lives at risk so that some people can enjoy short-term profits. In view of this, the beverage alcohol industry would be wise to avoid risking the pariah status that the continued support for this approach might invoke. Sensible policy should aim to eradicate harmful drinking, not drinking per se. In spite of this, the way to minimise alcohol problems is not simply to demonise and punish a minority. As indicated earlier in this book, the most obvious determinants of the level of alcohol problems are price and availability. The beverage alcohol industry should move beyond the unconvincing defence of ineffective policies. This would require a moral and logistic evolution to the honest acceptance of what the evidence *really* shows in relation to alcohol control policies. It would be wonderful if the industry, both in the UK and internationally, could rise to this challenge. Even so, many authorities have concluded that a business is simply that and that most industrial or commercial agencies function in self-interested, profit-seeking, amoral ways. The guru of monetarism, Milton Friedman, declared that it is the main aim of business to make money (Friedman 1970). Taken literally this apparently amoral view recalls the words of the reptilian character, Gordon Gecko, in the movie Wall Street: 'greed is good'.

There are of course, other views on business ethics (or lack of them). Ethical obligations such as decency, goodness, and social responsibility have also been acknowledged (Sternberg 1994, Cannon 1994, cited by Mullins 2005). One could also add honesty to this list. As Mullins has noted, intelligent self-interest should motivate a company or an industry to think of its social impact in the long-term as well as simply the short-term. In the case of industries that involve risks to public health or safety it is assumed that governments will take action to keep them in line in order to protect the population. The situation in the alcohol production industry has been transformed recently by the arrival of huge international agencies such as US based Anheuser-Busch and Belgian-based Interbrew (owner of Bass and Whitbread). It is reasonable to suppose that the social welfare of Britain may not be the most pressing concern of such organisations. The increasingly globalised nature of the industry makes it even more important that the UK government should act effectively to protect the British population from the harm caused by heavy drinking.

Price and availability are key issues that should not be ignored or down-played. Another key factor is the setting in which large numbers of young adults drink, especially in British towns and cities. As previously noted, we have created the perfect environment to foster heavy drinking and drunken-ness on a truly industrial scale. Town planning and licensing policy over the past decade at least have created concentrations of pubs and clubs that are a breeding ground for heavy drinking and public disorder. The alcohol policies covering the UK all include the obvious objective of reducing the adverse social and health consequences of heavy drinking. However, none have come to terms with the key issues of which ways are actually likely to do this.

A third way?

The 'Public Health approach' and 'harm minimisation' have sometimes been portrayed as being incompatible, even though they are justified by much the same evidence. Proponents of the two approaches have sometimes unflatter-ingly portrayed each other as 'extremists', 'alcohol terror mongers', 'stooges', or 'too friendly to the industry'. Personalities and professional rivalries explain some of this heat and venom. In fact, the evidence of which alcohol policies 'work' is fairly clear. There may even be a 'third way' of pursuing an effective alcohol policy.

Those who espouse the Public Health approach have sometimes overstated the case that problems such as liver disease always rise and fall in neat response to fluctuations in per capita alcohol consumption. The world is not quite that simple, so let's not pretend that it is. Those who, like the authors of this book, have advocated Harm minimisation have sometimes paid too little attention to the fact that if we really want to reduce alcohol problems, *a lot of people have to drink a lot less*. There is no logical or explicable reason why everyone needs to drink less, just those who drink heavily. Moderate drinkers would find it very strange if they were informed that their own drinking is dangerous. In spite of this, evidence shows that even many moderate drinkers sometimes have problems (e.g. Kreitman 1976). The most effective way to reduce the overall level of alcohol-related mayhem and tragedy is to put a cap on our national level of alcohol consumption. More drinking means more problems, less drinking means fewer problems.

The main aim of alcohol policy should be to stop people drinking heavily. The first step towards achieving this goal is for UK policies to be led by evidence and not by political expediency or commercial pressure. Policies should, in future, be mainly influenced by an honest determination to reduce the health and social problems associated with heavy drinking, whether in heavy episodic drinking sessions, 'binges', or as chronic high consumption.

The UK's leading health economist in the alcohol field is Professor Christine Godfrey of the University of York. She has calculated that 28% of drinks sold in the UK are consumed in 'binges' (Godfrey 2004). Since a lot of this is being sold in bars, it is clear that many bar staff are routinely and illegally selling drinks to intoxicated people.

The way forward?

The Government's suppressed 'Think Tank' report recommended using tax to curb alcohol problems back in 1979. These words were written at a time when per capita alcohol consumption and alcohol-related deaths were much lower than they are today. This has been shown in Figs 2.1, 3.7, and 3.8. The recommendations of the 'Think Tank' report have been echoed by reports from the Royal Colleges of Psychiatrists (1986), General Practitioners (1986) and Royal College of Physicians (1987), the Faculty of Public Health Medicine (1991), and the Academy of Medical Sciences (2004). These prestigious agencies have been disdainfully ignored by successive Conservative and Labour governments. These appear to have viewed effective alcohol control policy as an embarrassment that they prefer to ignore. This bipartisan political torpor has enabled both alcohol consumption and its related problems to keep on rising.

Britain is experiencing a level of heavy drinking that has not been evident since the nineteenth century. This drinking has been accompanied by a toll of adverse consequences that affect millions of people. As demonstrated by previous chapters, most of the major alcohol-related trends have been moving in the wrong direction, fostered by the increasing affordability of alcohol. Alcohol policy in different parts of the UK gives emphasis to measures that by themselves appear unlikely to make much difference to levels of either heavy drinking or its associated problems. The *Alcohol Harm Reduction Strategy for*

England does not even have specific targets, let alone much funding to back it up. However, a welcome additional £3.2 million for new initiatives to help identify and intervene early with people who have alcohol-related problems was announced by Public Health Minister Caroline Flint on November 1st, 2005 (Department of Health 2005).

The beverage alcohol industry is big, rich, and very powerful. It would appear that, so far as the major orientation of alcohol policy is concerned, it is also in the driver's seat. Sadly, it appears to be a very dangerous driver. The priorities of government are illustrated by the fact that far more civil servants are employed in relation to the production, distribution, and sale of alcohol than in relation to its health effects. Harrison and Tether (1987) reported that roughly ten times as many staff in HM Customs and Excise were involved with alcohol issues, compared with those (N=3.5 staff) in the Department of Health. This Department currently has an Alcohol Policy Team of five people with support staff. In contrast, Customs and Excise still has an Alcohol Strategy Team of over 300 people. These facts tell us much about the shape of national alcohol policy.

Industry influence appears to dictate the main shape of UK policy and renders it largely ineffective. The role of industry and its close links with government, particularly in the form of the DCMS, has become conspicuous in relation to recent events related to liquor licensing liberalisation in England and Wales. This legislation is being forced upon a people most of whom oppose it, with few defenders outside government and sections of the beverage alcohol industry. Available evidence suggests that this relaxation of licensing laws could exacerbate our existing alcohol problems. It could undermine the Government's wider agenda to reduce crime and disorder.

It is clear that the toll of alcohol problems in this country can only be reduced if alcohol consumption is reduced. Evidence suggests that any policy confined to measures solely targeted at heavy drinkers has scant chance of sustainable success. The most obvious and effective way to stop alcohol-related problems rising would be to prevent alcohol consumption in general rising by the use of tax to 'index-link' the affordability of alcohol in relation to household incomes. Policy should be designed to prevent any further rise in overall per capita alcohol consumption.

Furthermore, any serious policy intended to reduce the overall level of alcohol problems should go even further, by making alcohol less affordable. The price of alcoholic beverages could also usefully be adjusted following the Australian example, by imposing higher taxes on stronger beers and other beverages. As previously noted, this has been shown to reduce heavy drinking (Hall 2005a,b).

Another measure that could be used is to ensure that there are no further increases in either the number of licensed premises or bar opening hours. Licensing of such premises should, in future, be influenced by whether or not a locality needs extra premises within the overall framework of a local alcohol action plan. Such plans should be drawn up to cover all towns, cities, counties, or regions of the UK. These will require some radical measures in the interests of public health and safety. Some localities have far too many licensed premises. This probably encourages price wars between bars. Some of the existing urban bars are far too large. National legislation is required to ensure that all alcohol sold in bottles or cans within the UK is clearly labelled with a statement of the unit content.

It should be possible, even within the agenda of a health and safety-oriented alcohol policy, to cooperate with appropriate representatives of the beverage alcohol industry in relation to a number of important issues. These include the management of licensed premises, server training, codes of good practice, and alcohol advertising. The latter should become the subject of mandatory guidelines, independent adjudication and rigorous enforcement. It is not appropriate for the industry to retain its current influence in determining the overall shape of alcohol policy, notably in relation to price and availability. The industry has an obvious massive conflict of interest here that constitutes a very real threat to public health and safety (e.g. Stenius 2004).

Alcohol policy in all parts of the United Kingdom should go further than the Scottish approach that has some clear, but missed, targets. Policy should be designed to achieve significant and explicit reductions in heavy drinking and alcohol-related health and social problems. In the USA, raising the minimum legal drinking age achieved major important reductions in alcohol problems. In view of this, serious consideration should be given to raising the legal minimum age of alcohol consumption from five years of age to somewhere in the region of 16, 17, or 18 years of age. The American experience strongly suggests that this would achieve beneficial results. (Many people in Britain currently believe that it is already illegal for people to drink under the age of 18 years.) The authors believe that it would be unrealistic to raise the minimum drinking age to 21 years.

Crucially, the stabilisation and then the phased reduction of per capita alcohol consumption should be adopted as the foundation stone policy. This is needed to underpin and boost the impact of sustainable harm mini-misation measures. This would undoubtedly save a lot of harm.

Independent alcohol research in the UK is massively under-funded. (The Alcohol Education and Research Council has made an important contribution, but has very limited funds). UK alcohol research is at a much lower level than in several countries with much smaller populations. These include Canada, the Netherlands, and Sweden. This situation is unacceptable and should be quickly redressed. A new funding agency should be established to support a well-funded, long-term programme of independent social, psychological and medical research. The findings of such research should be published, not in the form of in-house reports, but through high quality peer-reviewed scientific journals. This research should include the design and evaluation of alcohol control policies. This agency *must* be completely free from influence by political and commercial interests.

In conclusion, we have lived with alcohol for a long time. As the social life and economic development of this country has ebbed and flowed, alcohol has been an important part of the picture. Most people drink and most of them enjoy doing so. Prohibition is not on the agenda, but a sustained reduction in alcohol-related disorder, crime, injury, illness, dependence, and premature mortality should be high on the agenda. The present government and its successors should be honest about what their alcohol policies are really primarily intended to achieve—to protect the public or to enable alcohol consumption and alcohol problems to continue rising unchecked. Public opinion might well back the protection of health and safety, even if this means paying more for a drink.

It is possible for the UK's constituent parts to adopt alcohol policies that are evidence-based, rational and effective. The dream of a relaxed, peaceful café society may not be utopian, provided our elected politicians have the wisdom and courage to introduce and sustain effective policies. These could neutralise the power of vested interests, transform the drinking environment and reclaim our town and city streets.

Bibliography

The following references were invaluable in the writing of this book. Many, though not all, have been cited in the text.

Abel, E. (1998) *Fetal Alcohol Abuse Syndrome*. New York: Plenum Press.

Academy of Medical Sciences (2004a) *Calling Time: the Nation's Drinking as a Health Issue*. London: Academy of Medical Sciences.

Academy of Medical Sciences (2004b) *Prime Minister's Strategy Unit Report on Alcohol Misuse*, (press release March 15th.). London: Academy of Medical Sciences.

Akhtar, P., Corbett, J., Currie, C., and Currie, D. (2004) *Scottish Schools Adolescent Lifestyle and Substance Use Survey (SALUS) National Report*. Norwich: TSO.

Alcohol Focus Scotland (2005) Holiday drink death, *Serve Wise*, Autumn, 3.

Alcoholics Anonymous Reviews (2005) Lager louts wreak havoc in Perth A&E, July 7th. http://www.aa-uk.org.uk/alcoholics-anonymous-reviews.

Alker, A. (2004) *The Big List: the Ultimate Guide to Alcohol Units*. Oldham: Hard Rain Productions.

Amt, E. (ed.) (1993) *Women's Lives in Medieval Europe*. London: Routledge.

Anderson, K. and Plant, M.A. (1996) Abstaining and carousing: Substance use among adolescents in the Western Isles of Scotland. *Drug and Alcohol Dependence*, 41, 196–9.

Andersson, B. (2002) *Oppna Rum: Om Undomarna, Staden Och Det Offenliga Livet* (Open Space: Youth, the City and Public life). Goteborg: Department of Social Work, Goteborg University.

Anonymous (1880) *Excuses to drink*. Temperance poem.

Annzai, Y. (2005) The relationship between alcohol consumption and health care utilisation among men in Japan: A reply to the Commentaries. *Addiction*, 100, 30.

Asthana, A. (2005) One bar, three hours—I was sold enough drink to kill me. *Observer*, October 24th, 8–9.

Aylin, P. (2004) Hospital admission trends. Presentation at *58th Alcohol Problems Research Symposium*, Kendal, March 2nd.

Babor, T., Caetano, R., Casswell, S., Edwards, G., Giesbrecht, N., Graham, K., *et al.* (2003) *Alcohol: No Ordinary Commodity*. Oxford: Oxford University Press.

Bach, P.J. and Shaefer, J.M. (1979) Tempo of country music and the rate of drinking in bars. *Journal of Studies on Alcohol*, 40, 1058–9.

Baer, J.S., Marlatt, A., and Mcmahon, R.J. (eds.) (1993) *Addictive Behaviors across the Life Span*. London: Sage.

Baggott, R. (1990) *Alcohol, Politics & Social Policy*. Avebury: Gower Publishing Company Ltd.

Bancroft, A., Wilson, S., Cunningham-Burley, S. Backett-Milburn, K., and Masters, H. (2004) *Parental Drug and Alcohol Use.* York: Joseph Rowntree Foundation.

Bandy, P. and President, P.A. (1983) Recent literature on drug abuse and prevention and mass media: focusing on youth, parents, women and elderly. *Journal of Drug Education,* 13, 255–1.

Barnard, M. (1999) Ladettes large it in Liverpool. *The Times,* Weekend, September 18th, 29.

Barnes-Powell, T. (1997) *Young Women and Alcohol: Issues of Pleasure and Power.* York: University of York

Barr, A. (1995) *Drink: an Informal Social History.* London: Bantam.

BBC (2003) website, September 17th.

BBC (2004) *Healthy Britain Survey,* August 9th.

BBC (2005) website, January 25th.

BBC (2005) Few pubs apply for late licences, BBC News Online, March 18th.

BBC (2005) *ASBO* boss in 'foul mouthed rant', July 6th.

BBC News Online (1999) World: South Asia drunken elephants trample village. October 21st. http:news.bbc.co.uk/2/hi/south_asia/482001.stm

BBC News Online (2002a) Drinking Law Shake-up Unveiled. November 15th. http://news.-bbc.co.uk_politics/2479609.stm

BBC News Online (2002b) Drinking Law Shake-up Unveiled November 15th. http://news.-bbc.co.uk/1/low/uk_politics/2479609.stm

BBC News Online (2003) Time called on drink ban rule, July 22nd. http://news.bbc.co.uk/1/low/wales/north_west/3086557.stm

BBC News Online (2004a) Government 'Sexed-down' Alcohol Report, June 7th. http://news.bbc.co.uk/go/pr/fr/-/1/hi/programmes/panorama/3767247.stm

BBC News Online (2005a) Fewer people visiting pubs. November 19th. http://news.-bbc.co.uk/1/hi/uk/4451706.stm

BBC News Online (2005b) Total smoking ban 'in ten years'. October 30th. http://news.-bbc.co.uk/2/hi/uk/news_politics/4387700.stm

BBC News Online (2005c) 'No Demand' For All-Day Drinking. 29th January. http://news.-bbc.co.uk/go/pr/fr/-/hi/uk/4217817.stm

BBC News Online (2005d) Alcohol 'as harmful as smoking' February 4th. http://news.-bbc.co.uk/2/hi/health/4232703.stm

BBC News Online (2005e) Drinks Law Shake-up Plan Defended. January 17th. http://news.bbc.co.uk/go/pr/fr/-/hi/uk_politics/4181551.stm

BBC News Online (2005f) NHS Fear Over 24-Hour Drink Plans. January 3rd. http://news.bbc.co.uk/go/pr/fr/-/hi/uk_politics/4142377.stm

BBC News Online (2005g) At-A-Glance: Drink Law Changes. January 21st. http://news.-bbc.co.uk/go/pr/fr/1/hi/uk_politics/4194741.stm

BBC News Online (2005h) Relaxing Reykjavik's Drinks Laws February 4th. http://news.-bbc.co.uk/go/pr/fr/-/1/hi/uk/4236121.stm

BBC News Online (2005i) A third of pubs to open longer. November 23rd. http://news.-bbc.co.uk/1/hi/uk_politics/4461888.stm

BBC News online (2005j) Asbo adviser mocks drink campaign. July 6th. http://news.-bbc.co.uk/1/hi/uk_politics/4654732.stm

BBC Wales (2005) Binge drinking survey. details provided by Davies, J. (personal communication April 12th).

Bennett, R., Tendler, S., and Ford, R. (2005) Late drinking law in danger as rebellion gathers pace. *Times*, August 11th, 1.

Bentham, M. and Temko, N. (2005) Lord Winston in tirade on drink laws, *Observer*, September 4th, 2.

Blackman, S. (1998) 'Poxy Cupid.' An ethnographic and feminist account of registered female youth culture, In T. Skelton and G. Valentine (eds.) *Cool Places: Geographies and Youth Cultures*, London: Routledge.

Bloomfield, K., *et al.* (2005) *Gender, Culture & Alcohol Problems: A Multi-National Study; Project Final Report*. Berlin: Charité Universitätsmedizin, Berlin.

Bloomfield, S. and Goodchild, S. (2005) Epidemic of liver disease hits women drinkers. *Independent on Sunday*, November 6th, 13.

Bonnie, R.J. (2003) Preface In: Bonnie, R.J. and O'Connell, M.E. (eds.) *Reducing Underage Drinking*. Washington, DC: The National Academies Press, pp. xv–xvi.

Bonnie, R.J. and O'Connell, M.E. (eds.) (2003) *Reducing Underage Drinking*. Washington, DC: The National Academies Press.

Booth, C. (1902) *Life and Labour of the People in London*. London: Macmillan and Co.

Bowcott, O. (2005) Rail police warn on licensing law. *Guardian*, August 25th, 10.

Boyd, G.M., Howard, J., and Zucker, R.A. (Eds.) (1995) *Alcohol Problems among Adolescents*. Hove: Lawrence Erlbaum Associates.

British Beer & Pub Association (2002) *Statistical Handbook*. London: British Beer & Pub Association.

British Beer & Pub Association (2005) *Point of Sale Promotions: Standards for the Management of Responsible Drinks Promotions Including Happy Hours*. London: British Beer & Pub Association.

British Market Research Bureau (2005) Public back extended drinking hours—but fear consequences. http:www.market researchworld.net/index.php?option=content&task-view&id=303.

Britton, A.R. (2001) *An Epidemiological Assessment of Alcohol and its Effect on Mortality in European Countries*. PhD thesis, London: University of London.

Brown, C. and Woolf, M. (2005) Labour retreats over round-the-clock drinking. *Independent*, August 11th, 6.

Brown, P. (2003) *Man Walks into a Pub*. London: Macmillan.

Bruun, K., Edwards, G., Lumio, M., Mäkelä, K., Pan, L., Popham R., *et al.* (1975) *Alcohol Control Policies in Public Health Perspective*. Helsinki: Finnish Foundation for Alcohol Studies.

Budd, T. (2003) *Alcohol-Related Assault: Findings from the British Crime Survey*. Online Report 35/03. London: Home Office.

Burnett, J. (1999) *Liquid Pleasures: A Social History of Drinks in Modern Britain*. London: Routledge.

Burns, L., Flaherty, B., Ireland, S., and Frances, M. (1995) Policing pubs: what happens to crime? *Drug and Alcohol Review*, 14, 369–5.

Butler, S. (2003) Paying the price for extended opening hours: A comment from Ireland. *Drugs: Education, Prevention & Policy* 10, 293–6.

Cabinet Office Prime Ministers' Strategy Unit (2003) *Alcohol Project: Interim Analytic Report.* London: Cabinet Office, 2003.

Cabinet Office Prime Minister's Strategy Unit (2004) *The Alcohol Harm Reduction Strategy for England.* London: Cabinet Office.

Camberwell Council on Alcoholism (1980) *Women and Alcohol.* London: Tavistock.

Cameron, D., Thomas, M., Madden, S., Thornton, C., Bergmark, A., Garretsen, H., *et al.* (2000) Intoxicated across Europe: In search of meaning. *Addiction Research* 8, 233–42.

Campaign for Real Ale (2005) CAMRA's survey on licensing hours. *Ale,* Spring **309**.

Cannon, T. (1994) *Corporate Responsibility.* London: Pitman.

Carter H. (1919) *The Control of the Drink Trade in Britain: A Contribution to National Efficiency during the Great War 1915–1918.* London, Longman: Green and Co.

Carvel, J. (2005a) Britons drink more alcohol as French cut intake. *Guardian,* August 24th, 7.

Carvel, J. (2005b) Girls more likely to smoke and get drunk. *Guardian,* August 27th, 6.

Cavan, S. (1966) *Liquor License: An Ethnography of Bar Behavior.* Chicago: Aldine.

Central Policy Review Staff (1979) *Alcohol Policies in the United Kingdom.* Stockholm: Sociologiska Institutionen, Stockholms Universitat (printed in 1982).

Chaloupka, F.J. and Weschler, H. (1995) *The Impact of Price, Availability, and Alcohol Control Policies on Binge Drinking in College.* Cambridge, Massachusetts: National Bureau of Economic Research, Working Paper 3831.

Chaloupka, F.J., Saffer, H., and Grossman, M. (1991) *Alcohol Control Policies and Motor Vehicle Fatalities.* Cambridge, Massachusetts: National Bureau of Economic Research.

Chaloupka, F.J., Grossman, M. and Saffer, H. (1998) Effects of price on the consequences of alcohol use and abuse. In: Galanter, M. (ed.) *Recent Developments in Alcoholism, Vol 14, The Consequences of Alcoholism.* Chicago: University of Chicago Press.

Channel Four (2005) Poll reveals appalling attitudes to rape (survey for Amnesty International). November 21st. http://www.channel4.com/news/content/newsstorypage.jsp?id=1875378

Chapman, D. (2005) Huge slump in public support for 24-hour pubs. *Daily Mail* January 26th.

Chatterton, P. and Hollands, R. (2003) *Urban Nightscapes: Youth Cultures, Pleasure Spaces and Corporate Power.* London: Routledge.

Chikritzhs, T. and Stockwell, T. (2002) The impact of later trading hours for Australian public houses (hotels) on levels of violence. *The Journal of Studies on Alcohol,* **63**, 591–9.

Chrisafis, A. and Carvel, J. (2005) Northern Ireland smoking ban puts pressure on England to toe the line. *Guardian,* October 5th, 4.

Claes L., Vandereycken W., and Vertommen H. (2005) Self-care versus self-harm: Piercing, tattooing and self-injury in eating disorders. *European Eating Disorders Review* **13**, 11–18.

Clark H. and Carnegie E. (2003) *She Was Aye Working.* Oxford: White Cockade Publishing.

Clark, P. (1983) *The English Alehouse: A Social History 1200–1830.* London: Longman.

Clark, P. (1988) The 'Mother Gin' controversy in early eighteenth century England. *Transactions of the Royal Society,* **38**, 63–84.

Clayson, C. (1973) *Report of the Departmental Committee on Scottish Licensing Law.* Edinburgh: HMSO.

Coate, D. and Grossman, M. (1988) Effects of alcoholic beverage prices and legal drinking age on youth alcohol use. *Journal of Law and Economics*, 31, 145–71.

Coates, S., Tendler, S. and Sherman, J. (2005) Pubs ready to party in face of objectors who never stood a chance. *Times*, November 21st, 16.

Cohen, S. (1972) *Folk Devils and Moral Panics*. London: MacGibbon and Kee.

Collins, J.J. jnr. (ed.) (1982) *Drinking and Crime*. London: Tavistock.

Colorado Alcohol and Drug Abuse Division (1990) *Analysis of Selected Alcohol and Drug Related Risk Factors for the 634 Counties and Statewide Average, 1986–1990*. Denver, Colorado: Colorado Alcohol and Drug Abuse Division.

Commission on Liquor Licensing (2003) *Final Report* April 2nd http://www.justice.ie/80256E010039C5AF/vWeb/pcJUSQ629CYR-en

Cooke, P.J. (1981) The effect of liquor taxes on drinking, cirrhosis and auto faculities. In Moore, M. and Gerstein D. (eds) *Alcohol and Public Policy*, Washington, DC, National Academy of Sciences.

Cooke, P.J. and Moore, M.J. (1993) Drinking and schooling. *Journal of Health Economics*, 12, 411–29.

Cooke, P.J. and Moore, M. (1993) Taxation of alcoholic beverages. In: Hilton, M.E. and Bloss, G. (eds.) *Economics and the Prevention of Alcohol-Related Problems*, Research Monograph No 25, NIH publication No. 93-3513. Rockville Maryland: National Institute on Alcohol Abuse and Alcoholism, pp.33–58.

Cooke, P.J. and Tauchen, E. (1982) The effect of liquor taxes on heavy drinking. *Bell Journal of Economics* 13: 379–390.

Cracknell, D. (2005) No drinking on buses or trains. *Sunday Times*, October 30th, 1.

Crombie, I., Irvine, L., Elliott, L., and Wallace, H. (2005) *Public Health Policy on Alcohol*. Dundee: University of Dundee/NHS Health Scotland.

Cummins, J.C. (1993) *Licensing Law in Scotland*. Edinburgh: Butterworths/Law Society of Scotland.

Dáil Éireann (2000) The Intoxicating Liquor Bill 2000, volume 519. May 25th. http://historical-debates.oireachtas.ie/D/0519/D.0519.200005250005.html

Daily Mail (2005a) Boozing Britain: Another Cover-up. *Daily Mail*, January 18th, 8–9.

Daily Mail (2005b) Cherie's dad pours scorn on licencing laws. November 23rd, P. 4.

Datamonitor (2004) *New Trends in Young Adults' Alcoholic Drinks Occasions*. London: Datamonitor.

Davies, J.B. and Stacey, B. (1972) *Teenagers and Alcohol*. London: HMSO.

De Crespigny, C. (2001) Young women, pubs and safety. In: Williams, P. (ed.) (2001) *Alcohol, Young Persons and Violence*. Canberra: Australian Institute of Criminology, pp.31–46.

Deehan, A. (1999) *Alcohol and Crime: Taking Stock*. London: Policing and Reducing Crime Unit, Home Office.

Delgado, M. (2005) Blair aide in battle to stop his local extending opening hours, *Mail on Sunday*, September 4th, 13.

Department of Culture, Media and Sport (2002). Tessa Jowell praises pub industry and promises reform. Press notice, April 25th.

Department of Culture, Media and Sport (2004) *Guidance Issued under Section 182 of the Licensing Act 2003*. London: Department of Culture, Media and Sport.

Department of Culture, Media and Sport (2005) *Licensing Act 2003*. http://www.culture.-gov/uk/alcohol_entertainment/licensing_act.htm

Department of the Environment (2005) *Family Food—Expenditure and Food Survey*. London: Department of the Environment.

Department of Health (1999) *Drinking: Adults' Behaviour and Knowledge in 1998: A Report on Research for the Department of Health Using the ONS Omnibus Survey*. London: Stationery Office.

Department of Health (2001) *Annual Report of the Chief Medical Officer*. London: Department of Health.

Department of Health (2005) Boost for alcohol treatment provision with publication of programme of improvement. November 1st, press release number 2005/0375.

Department of Health, Social Services and Public Safety (Northern Ireland) (2000) *Strategy for Reducing Alcohol-Related Harm*. Belfast: Department of Health, Social Services and Public Safety.

Dickson-Wright, C. (2005). Will nobody learn the lessons of Scotland? *Daily Mail*, January 18th, 8.

Dight, S. (1976) *Scottish Drinking Habits*. London: HMSO.

Dillon, P. (2003) *The Much Lamented Death of Madam Geneva*. London: Justin, Charles and Company.

Dilulio, J.J. (1995) *Broken Bottles, Liquor, Disorder and Crime in Wisconsin*. Milwaukee, Wisconsin: Wisconsin Policy Research Institute.

Disley, J. (2005a) An alcopops addict at 10, *Daily Mirror*, November 1st, 1, 5.

Disley, J. (2005b) Killed by 40 minute booze binge, *Daily Mirror*, August 25th, 1, 11.

Donnelly, N. and Briscoe, S. (2005) Intelligence led regulation of licensed premises, In: Stockwell, T., Gruenewald., P.J., Toumbourou, J.W. and Loxley, W. (eds.) (2005) *Preventing Harmful Substance Abuse*. Chichester: Wiley, pp.257–64.

Doward, J. (2005) Police fear chaos over pub hours. *Observer*, March 20th, 6.

Doward, J and Asthana, A. (2005) New poll boosts demand for total pub smoking ban. *Observer*, September 18th, 7.

Doward, J., Hinsliff, G. and Temko, N. (2005) Health watchdog warns on drink law. *Observer*, November 20th, 3.

Downing, S. (2005) letter. *The Guardian* November 1st. p. 31.

Drummond, D.C. (2000) UK Government announces first major relaxation in the alcohol licensing laws for nearly a century: drinking in the UK goes 24–7. *Addiction* 95, 997–8.

Drummond, D.C. (2004) An alcohol strategy for England: The good, the bad and the ugly, *Alcohol & Alcoholism* 39, 377–9.

Duffy, J.W., Plant, M.A. (1986) Scotland's liquor licensing changes: An assessment. *British Medical Journal*, 292, 36–9.

Edwards, G. (2000) *Alcohol: The Ambiguous Molecule*. Harmondsworth: Penguin.

Edwards, G., Anderson, P., Babor, T., Casswell, S., Ferrence, R. Giesbrecht, N., *et al.* (1995) *Alcohol Policy and the Public Good*. Oxford: Oxford University Press.

Egginton, R., Williams, L. and Parker, H. (2002) Going out drinking: The centrality of heavy alcohol used in English adolescents' leisure time and poly substance taking, *Journal of Substance Use*, 7, 125–35.

Elkind, D. (1967) Egocentrism in adolescence. *Child Development*, **30**, 1025–34.

Elkind, D. (1984) Teenage thinking: Implications for health care. *Paediatric Nursing*, 10, 383–5.

Elliott, F. (2005) Cabinet war over smoking ban. *Independent on Sunday*, October 23rd, 5.

Encylopaedia Brittanica (1911) London: Encylopaedia Brittanica, p. 22.

Engineer, R., Phillips, A., Thompson, J., and Nicholls, J. (2003) *Drunk and Disorderly: A Qualitative Study of Binge Drinking among 18 to 24 Year Olds*. Home Office Research Study Number 262, London: Home Office.

Erroll of Hale (1972) *Report of the Departmental Committee on Liquor Licensing*. London: HMSO.

Faculty of Public Health Medicine (1991) *Alcohol and the Public Health*. London: Macmillan.

Fagan, J. (1993) Set and setting revisited: Influences of alcohol and illicit drugs on the social context of violent events. In: Martin, S.E. (ed.) *Alcohol and Interpersonal Violence: Fostering Multidisciplinary Perspectives*. Rockville, Maryland: National Institute of Health, 224, 160–92.

Farrell, S., Manning, W.G. and Finch, M.D. (2003) Alcohol dependence and the price of alcoholic beverages. *Journal of Health Economics*, 22, 117–47.

Ferguson, S. (1975) *Drink*. London: Batsford.

Firth (1880) *Brandy: What it is, what it does, what it cannot do*. Read at the Autumn Conference of British Temperance Association, Bristol, November 1880

Ford, R. and Tendler, S. (2005) New drinking laws will end in violence, warn judges. *The Times*, August 10th, 1–2.

Ford, R., Sherman, J., and Rumbelow, H. (2005) Police powerless to stop late-night drinking without proof of disorder, *The Times*, August 24th, p6.

Fossey, E. (1994) *Growing up with Alcohol*. London: Tavistock/Routledge.

Foster, D. (2005a) Sober facts (letter) *Guardian*, August 20th, 19.

Foster, D. (2005b) Drinking laws will be hard to swallow, (letter) *Guardian*, October 1st, 31.

Foster, J. (2003) Extended alcohol licensing hours in England and Wales: There will be a large price to pay. *Drugs: Education, Prevention and Policy*, 10, 285–7.

Foxcroft, D.R., Lister-Sharp, D. and Lowe, G. (1997) Alcohol misuse prevention for young people: A systematic review reveals methodological concerns and lack of reliable evidence of effectiveness. *Addiction*, 92, 531–7.

Foxcroft, D., Ireland, D., Lister-Sharp, D.J., and Breen, R. (2003) Longer-term primary prevention for alcohol misuse in young people: A systematic review, *Addiction* 98, 397–411.

French, R.V. (1890) *Nineteen Centuries of Drink in England*. London: National Temperance Publication Depot.

Friedman, M. (1970) The social responsibility of business is to increase its profits, *New York Times Magazine*, September 13th, 122–6.

Friedman, L.A. and Kimbal, A.W. (1986) Coronary heart disease motality and alcohol consumption in Framingham. *American Journal of Epidemiology*, 124: 481–489.

Garretsen, H. (2003) Alcohol across Europe presentation at *Durham 2003*, Addictions Forum residential event, Durham Castle, September 26th.

Gibb, F., de Bruxelles, S., and Coates, S. (2005) Women can't claim rape when drunk, judge rules, *Times*, November 24th, 1.

Gibbons, E. (2001) *All Beer and Skittles: A Short History of Inns and Taverns*. London: The National Trust.

Gilmore, I. (2004) The medical effects of heavy drinking, presentation at international conference. *Binge Drinking: Problems & Responses*, Bristol, November 26th.

Gill, A.A. (2005) *The Angry Island*. London: Orion.

Gmel, G (2005) Personal communication.

Goddard, E., Plant, M.A. Plant, M.L., Davidson, I., and Garretsen, H. (2000) Drinking patterns In: Plant, M.A. and Cameron, I. (eds.) *The Alcohol Report.* London: Free Association Books, pp.56–78.

Godfrey, C. (1997) Can tax be used to minimise harm? A health economist's perspective, In: Plant, M.A., Single, E. and Stockwell, T. (eds.) *Alcohol: Minimising the Harm: What Works?* London: Free Association Books, pp.29–42.

Godfrey, C. (2004) The economics of binge drinking, paper presented at international conference on *Binge Drinking: Problems & Responses,* Bristol, UK, November 26th.

Goossens, L., Beyers, W., Emmen, M. and van Aken, M. (2002) The imaginary audience and personal fable: Factor analyses and concurrent validity of the "new look" measures, *Journal of Research on Adolescence.* 12, 193–215.

Graham H.G. (1950) *The Social Life of Scotland in the Eighteenth Century.* London: Adam & Charles Black.

Graham, K. (1985) Determinants of heavy drinking and drinking problems: the contribution of the bar environment, In: Single, E. and Storm, T. (eds.) *Public Drinking and Public Policy.* Toronto: Addiction Research Foundation, pp.71–84.

Graham, K. and Homel, R. (1997) Creating safer bars, In: Plant, M.A., Single, E. and Stockwell, T. (eds.) *Alcohol: Minimising the Harm: What Works?* London: Free Association Books, pp.171–92.

Graham, K., LaRoque, L., Yetman, R., Ross, T.J., and Guistra, E. (1980) Aggression and barroom environments, *Journal of Studies on Alcohol,* 41, 277–92.

Graham, K., Plant, M.L., and Plant, M.A. (2004) Alcohol, gender and partner aggression: A general population study of British adults. *Addiction Research and Theory* 12, 385–401.

Greenaway, J. (2003) *Drink and British Politics since 1830: A Study in Policy Making.* Basingstoke: Palgrave Macmillan.

Greenfield, T.K. (1997) Warning labels: Evidence on harm reduction from long-term American surveys, In: Plant, M.A., Single, E. and Stockwell, T. (eds.) *Alcohol: Minimising the Harm: What Works?* London: Free Association Books, pp.105–25.

Greenfield, T.K. and Giesbrecht, N.A. (2005) Views of alcohol control policies in the 2000 National Alcohol Survey: What news for alcohol policy in the US and its states, (unpublished).

Greenfield, T.K., Johnson, S.P., and Giesbrecht, N.A. (2004) Public opinion on alcohol policy: A review of U.S. research. *Contemporary Drug Problems,* 31, 759–90.

Grønbæk, M., Deis, A., Sørensen, T., Becker, U., Schnor, P., and Jensen, G. (1995) Mortality associated with moderate intakes of wine, beer, or spirits. *British Medical Journal,* 310, 1165–9.

Grossman, M., Coate, D., and Arluck, G.M. (1987) Price sensitivity of alcoholic beverages in the United States: Youth alcohol consumption. In: Holder, H. (ed.) *Advances in Substance Abuse: Behavioural and Biological Research. Control Issues in Alcohol Abuse Prevention: Strategies for States and Communities,* Greenwich, Connecticut: JAI Press, pp.169–98.

Grossman, M., Chaloupka, F.J., and Sirtalan, I. (1998) An empirical analysis of alcohol addiction: Results from the Monitoring the Future panels, *Economic Inquiry,* 36, 39–48.

Guardian, (2005a) Call time on licensing changes, (Editorial). *Guardian,* September 22nd, 34.

Guardian (2005b) On the spot drink fines. *Guardian*, April 2nd, 10.

Guardian (2005c) Pub food to go in light of ban, *Guardian*, September 7th, 9.

Hackwood, F. (1910/1985) *Inns, Ales and Drinking Customs of Old England*. Simsbury, Connecticut: Bracken Books.

Haines, B. and Graham, K. (2005) Violence prevention in licensed premises, In: Stockwell, T., Gruenewald., P.J., Toumbourou, J.W. and Loxley, W. (eds.) *Preventing Harmful Substance Abuse*, Chichester: Wiley, pp.163–76.

Hall, W. (2005a) Alcohol misuse, public health and public policy, *British Medical Journal* 331, 1343–4.

Hall, W. (2005b) British drinking: A suitable case for treatment? (editorial). *British Medical Journal* 331, 527–8.

Hansard (1995) Budget speech by Chancellor of the Exchequer, Kenneth Clarke, column 1065.

Hansard (2005) Debate on licensing, October 24th, column 89.

Harding, L. (2005) Drunken elks attack old people's home, *Guardian*, November 11th, 4.

Harnett, R., Thom, B., Herring, R. and Kelly, M. (2000) Alcohol in transition: Towards a model of young men's drinking styles, *Journal of Youth Studies* 3, 61–77.

Harris, C. (2005) Our city centres are abandoned to drunk, noisy louts. *Times*, August 10th, 2.

Harrison, B.N. (1971) *Drink and the Victorians*. London: Faber and Faber.

Harrison, L. and Tether, P. (1987) The coordination of UK policy on alcohol and tobacco: the significance of organisational networks. *Policy and Politics*, 15, 77–90.

Hauritz, M., Homel, R., McIlwain, G., Burrows, T., and Townsley, M. (1998) Reducing violence in licensed venues through community safety action projects: The Queensland experience. *Contemporary Drug Problems*, 25, 511–51.

Hawthorne, G., Garrard, J. and Dunt, D. (1995) Does Life Education's drug education programme have a heath benefit? *Addiction*, 90, 205–16.

Health Promotion Agency for Northern Ireland (2000) *The Health Behaviour of School Children in Northern Ireland: A Report on the 1997/98 Survey*. Belfast: Health Promotion Agency for Northern Ireland.

Health Promotion Agency for Northern Ireland (2002) *Adult Drinking Patterns in Northern Ireland*. Belfast: Health Promotion Agency for Northern Ireland.

Health Promotion Agency for Northern Ireland (undated) *Attitudes and Behaviour of Young Adult Drinkers in Northern Ireland*: Belfast: Health Promotion Agency for Northern Ireland.

Heath, D. (ed.) (1995) *International Handbook on Alcohol and Culture*. Westport, Connecticut: Greenwood Press.

Heather, N. (1997) Psychosocial treatment approaches and findings from Project Match. In: Plant, M.A. and Cameron, D. (eds.) *The Alcohol Report*. London, Free Association Books, pp. 154–77.

Hetherington, P. (2005) Pressure mounts to delay 24 hour drinking, *Guardian*, January 18th, 4.

Hetherington, P. and Bowers, S. (2005) Time Called on Happy Hour Drinking in City Hotspots. *Guardian* February 7th. http://www.guardian.co.uk/print/0,3858,5120987-103690,00.html

Henstridge, J., Homel, R. and MacKay, P. (1997) *The Long-term Effects of Random Breath Testing in Four Australian States: A Time Series Analysis.* Canberra: Federal Office of Road Safety.

Hey, V. (1986) *Patriarchy and Pub Culture.* London: Tavistock.

Hibell, B., Andersson, B., Bjarnason, T., Kokkevi, A., Morgan, M. and Narusk, A. (1997) *The 1995 ESPAD Report: Alcohol and Other Drug Use amongst Students in 26 European Countries.* Stockholm: Swedish Council for Information on Alcohol and Other Drugs.

Hibell, B., Andersson, B., Balakireva, O., Bjarnasson, T. Kokkevi, A., and Morgan, M. (2001) *The 1999 ESPAD Report: Alcohol and Other Drug Use among Students in 30 European Countries.* Stockholm: Swedish Council for Information on Alcohol and Other Drugs.

Hibell, B., Andersson, B., Bjarnasson, T. Ahlström, S., Balakireva, O., Kokkevi, A. *et al.* (2004) *The 2003 ESPAD Report: Alcohol and Other Drug Use among Students in 30 European Countries.* Stockholm: Swedish Council for Information on Alcohol and Other Drugs.

Hickley, M. (2005a) Booze blackmailers: Clarke blasts pub chiefs in new licensing fiasco. *Daily Mail,* September 28th, 13.

Hickley, M. (2005b) How drink helped the rise in violent crime. *Daily Mail,* October 21st, 15.

Hickley, M. (2005c) 24-hour booze at the checkout. *Daily Mail,* August 25th, 1–10.

Hickley, M. and Mills, J. (2005) The great 24-hour drink con. *Daily Mail,* November 23rd, 8.

Hickman, M. (2005) Supermarkets to face inquiry over alcohol sales to children. *Independent,* November 16th, 21.

Hilton, M. and Kaskutas, L.A. (1991) Changes in public support for warning labels on alcoholic beverage containers. *British Journal of Addiction,* 86, 1323–33.

Hingson, R.W. and Kenkel, D. (2004) Social, health and economic consequences of underage drinking. In: *National Research Council and Institute of Medicine: Reducing Underage Drinking: a Collective Responsibility.* Committee on Developing a Strategy to Reduce and Prevent Underage Drinking, Division of Behavioural and Social Sciences and Education, Washington, DC: The National Academies Press.

Hingson, R., Berson, J. and Dowley, K. (1997) Interventions to reduce college student drinking and related health and social problems, In: Plant, M.A., Single, E. and Stockwell, T. (eds.) *Alcohol: Minimising the Harm: What Works?* London: Free Association Books, pp. 143–70.

Hinscliffe, G. (2005) New ads to tackle binge drink culture, *Observer,* August 14th, 2.

Hinscliffe, G. and Asthana, A. (2005) Drink Giants plans to fuel binge Britain. *Observer,* October 23rd, 1–2.

Hinscliffe, G. and Doward, J. (2005) Total ban on smoking as Blair gives way, *Observer,* October 9th, p1.

Hobbs, D. (2002) The night time economy. In: Macara, A. (ed.) *100% Proof: Research for Action on Alcohol.* London: Alcohol Concern, pp. 58–61.

Hollands, R. (1995) *Friday Night, Saturday Night: Youth Identification in the Post-Industrial City.* Newcastle upon Tyne: Department of Sociology, University of Newcastle University.

Hollands, R. and Chatterton, P. (2001) *Changing our Toon: Youth, Nightlife and Urban Change in Newcastle.* Newcastle: University of Newcastle.

Home Office (2003) *Drinking, Crime and Disorder* (Findings 185). London: Home Office.

Home Office (2004) *Arrests for Notifiable Offences and the Operation of Certain Police Powers under PACE.* Statistical Bulletin 18/04, London: Home Office.

Home Office Online (2005) Drug-assisted sexual assault, http://www.homeoffice.gov.uk/crime/sexualoffences/drug_assisted.html

Homel, R., Carseldine, D. and Kearns, I. (1988) Drink driving counter-measures in Australia. *Alcohol, Drugs and Driving,* 4, 113–44.

Homel, R. and Clark, J. (1994) The prediction and prevention of violence in pubs and clubs. *Crime Prevention Studies,* 3, 10–46.

Homel, R., Tomsen, S. and Thommeny, J. (1992) Public drinking and violence: Not just an alcohol problem. *Journal of Drug Issues,* 222, 679–97.

Homel, R., Hauritz, M., Wortley, R., Clark, J., and Carvolth, R. (1994) *The Impact of the Surfers' Paradise Safety Action Project: Key Findings of the Evaluation.* Griffith University: Centre for Crime Policy and Public Safety.

Hope, J. (2005) One in four is classed as a binge drinker, *Daily Mail,* October 27th, 29.

House of Commons (1852–1854) *Reports of the Select Committee of the House of Commons on Public Houses and Morals* (The Villiers Committee). London: House of Commons.

House of Commons (1896–1898) *Royal Commission on the Liquor Licensing Laws* (The Peel Committee). London: House of Commons.

House of Commons Home Affairs Committee (2005) *Anti-Social Behaviour.* Fifth report of session, Volume 1, April 5th.

Hunt, J., and Satterlee, S. (1987) Cohesion and division: Drinking in an English pub. *Man,* 21, 521–37.

Hutt, C. (1973) *The Death of the English Pub.* London: Hutchinson.

Iredale W. (2005) New law may only delay pub violence, *Sunday Times,* November 6th, 1–7.

Jahoda, G. and Cramond, J. (1972) *Children and Alcohol,* London: HMSO.

Jarvis, M. (2004) Personal communication.

Jeffs, B. and Saunders, W. (1983) Minimising alcohol-related offences by enforcement of the existing legislation. *British Journal of Addiction* 78, 67–78.

Jernigan, D.H. and Mosher, J. (2005) Editors' introduction: Alcohol marketing and youth-public health perspectives. *Journal of Public Health Policy* 26, 287–91.

Johnston, B. (2004) Anglo Saxon drink binges introduce Italy to lager louts. *Telegraph News,* December 18th.

Johnston, J. (2005) Scots Attack 24-Hour Drinking Reform Plan *The Sunday Herald,* January 16th. http://www.sundayherald.com/print47161

Johnston, L., O'Malley, P.M. Bachman, J.G. and Schulenberg, J.E. (2004) *Monitoring the Future: National Survey Results on Drug Use 1975–2003, Volume I: Secondary School Students.* Bethesda, Maryland: National Institute on Drug Abuse.

Johnston, P. (2005) 70,000 pubs and clubs call an end to time, *Daily Telegraph,* November 24th, 1.

Jowell, T. (2005a) I hope that Mrs May won't take a tipple after 11pm. *The Independent on Sunday,* August 28th, 21.

Jowell, T. (2005b) A start in fixing our problems. *Daily Mirror,* November 23rd, 10.

Kalb, M. (1975) The myth of alcoholism prevention. *Preventive Medicine,* 4, 404–16.

Kaskutas, L.A. (1993) Changes in public attitudes toward alcohol control policies since warning labels mandate of 1989. *Journal of Public Policy and Marketing,* 12, 30–7.

Kaukinen, C. (2002) Adolescent victimization and problem drinking. *Violence and Victims*, 17, 669–89.

Keeble, N.H. (1994) *A Cultural Identity of Seventeenth Century Woman: A Reader*, London: Routledge.

Kessel, N. and Walton, H. (1965) *Alcoholism*. Harmondsworth: Pelican.

Kettle, M (2003) My Name is Britain, and I have a drink problem *Guardian*, May 31st. http://society.guardian.co.uk/drugsandalcohol/comment/o,8146,967666,00.html

Kinder, B.N., Pape, N.E., and Walfish, S. (1980) Drug and alcohol education programs: a review of outcome studies. *International Journal of the Addictions*, 15, 1035–56.

King E. (1993) *The Hidden History of Glasgow's Women*. Edinburgh and London: Mainstream Publishing.

Kirkham, S. (2005) Women warned after city is hit by rape gang. *Guardian*, August 11th, 4.

Klatsky, A.L. and Armstrong, M.A. (1993) Alcohol use, other traits, and risk of unnatural death. *Alcoholism: Clinical and Experimental Research*, 17, 1156–62.

Klatsky, A.L., Armstrong, M.A., and Friedman, G.D. (1986) Relation of alcoholic beverage use to subsequent coronary artery disease hospitalization. *American Journal of Cardiology*, 58, 710–14.

Klepp, K.I., Schmid, L.A., and Murray, D.M. (1996) Effects of increased minimum drinking age law on drinking and driving behaviour among adolescents. *Addiction Research*, 4: 237–244.

Kneale, J. (1999) A problem of supervision: Moral geographies of the nineteenth century British public house. *Journal of Historical Geography* 25, 333–48.

Kneale, J. (2001) The place of drink: temperance and the public, 1856–1914. *Social and Cultural Geography*, 2, 43–59.

Kreitman, N. (1976) Alcohol consumption and the preventive paradox. *British Journal of Addiction*, 81, 353–63.

Ledoux, S., Miller, P., Choquet, M. and Plant, M.A. (2002) Family structure, parent-child relationships, and alcohol and other drug use among teenagers in France and the United Kingdom. *Alcohol & Alcoholism*, 37, 52–60.

Lees, L. (1993) Urban renaissance and the street: Spaces of control and contestation, In: Fyfle, N.R. (ed.) *Images of the Street: Planning, Identity and Control in Public Space.* London: Routledge.

Leigh, D., Evans, R., and Gould, M. (2005) Relatively cheaper alcohol fuels big increase in consumption since 1979. *Guardian*, November 17th, 9.

Lemmens, P.H., Vaeth, P.A.C., and Greenfield, T.K. (1999) Coverage of beverage alcohol issues in the print media in the US, 1985–1991. *American Journal of Public Health*, 89, 1555–60.

Leppard, D., and Winnett, R. (2005) Blunkett's Anger over Drink Laws *Times Online* January 16th. http://www.timesonline.co.uk/printFriendly/0,,1-523-1442611-523,00.html

Leung, S.F. and Phelps, C.E. (1993) My kingdom for a drink . . . ? A review of estimates of the price sensitivity of demand for alcoholic beverages. In: Hilton, M.E. and Bloss, G. (eds.) *Economics and the Prevention of Alcohol-Related Problems*, Rockville, Maryland: National Institute on Alcohol Abuse and Alcoholism, Research Monograph No 25, US Department of Health and Human Services, pp.1–341.

Lewis, J. (2005a) Residents' revolt: Government forced to water down new drinks laws after fierce pressure from householders. *Mail on Sunday*, September 18th, 7.

Lewis, J. (2005b) Prescott covering up the effects of 24-hour drinking. *Mail on Sunday*, November 20th, 8.

Liberal Democrats Online (2005) House of Lords—Licensing Act 2003 (Second Appointed day) Order 2005. http://www.libdems.org.uk.parliammnet/licensing-act-delay-binge-drinking-crime-1441

Light, R. (1999) *The Concept of Need in Liquor Licensing*. Bristol: Faculty of Law: University of the West of England.

Light, R. (2000) Liberalising liquor licensing law. *New Law Journal*, **150**, 6941.

Light, R. (2003) Open all hours? *Solicitors Journal*, **147**, 842.

Light, R. (2005) The Licensing Act 2003: Liberal constraint? *Law Review* **68**, 268–85.

Lilywight, B. (1963) *London Coffee Houses*. London: Allen and Unwin.

Linklater, M. (2005) Last orders for licences: Yet another fiasco in the great legislation binge. *The Times*, August 24th, 19.

Lipton, R., and Gruenwald, P. (2002) Spatial dynamics of violence and alcohol outlets. *Journal of Studies on Alcohol*, **63**, 187–95.

Lister, S., Hobbs, D., Hall, S., and Winslow, S. (2000) Violence in the night-time economy; bouncers: The reporting, recording and prosecution of assaults. *Policing and Society*, **10**, 383–402.

Lopez-Claros, A. and Zahidi, S. (2005) *Women's Empowerment: Measuring the Global Gender Gap*. Geneva: World Economic Forum.

Loretto, W. (1994) Youthful drinking in Northern Ireland and Scotland: Preliminary results from a comparative study. *Drugs, Education, Prevention and Policy*, **1**, 143–52.

Ludbrook, A., Godfrey, C., Wyness, L., Parrott, S., Haw, S., Napper, M. *et al.* (2001) *Effective and Cost-Effective Measures to Reduce Alcohol Misuse in Scotland*. Edinburgh: Scottish Executive.

Lupton, M.J. (1979) Ladies' entrance: Women and bars. *Feminist Studies*, **5**, 571–88.

Luty, J. (2005) UK alcohol policy-pure genius, (editorial), *Psychiatric Bulletin*, **29**, 410–12.

MacAndrew, C. and Edgerton, R.B. (1969) *Drunken Comportment: A Social Explanation*. Chicago: Aldine.

Macdonald, S. (1994) Whisky, Women and the Scottish Drink Problem. A View from the Highlands, In: McDonald, M. (ed.) *Gender, Drink and Drugs: Cross Cultural Perspectives on Women*. Oxford/Providence USA: Berg.

Macdonell, H. (2005) Licensing bill leads to shambles in a former brewery. *Scotsman*, November 17th, 3.

MacLaren, A.A. (1976) *Social Class in Scotland Past and Present*. Edinburgh: John Donald Publishers.

MacLean, C. (2003) *Scotch Whisky. A Liquid History*, London: Cassell Illustrated.

Maguire, M. and Nettleton H. (2003) *Reducing Alcohol-Related Violence and Disorder: An Evaluation of the TASC Project*. London: Home Office (Research Study 265).

Mäkelä, P., Rossow, I., and Tryggvesson, K. (2002) Who Drinks More and Less When Policies Change? The evidence from 50 years of Nordic studies. In Room R. (ed.) *The Effects of Nordic Alcohol Policies: what happens to drinking and harm when alcohol controls change?* NAD Publication 42, Helsinki, Finland, pp.17–70.

Malcolm, E. (1986) *Ireland Sober, Ireland Free: Drink and Temperance in Nineteenth-Century Ireland* Dublin. Gill and MacMillan.

Manchester Online (2004) Underage alcohol sales crackdown, September 17th, http://www.manchesteronline.co.uk/news/s/130/130742_underage_alcohol_sales_crac

Manning, W.G., Blumberg, L. and Moulton, L.H. (1995) The demand for alcohol: The differential response to price. *Journal of Health Economics,* 14, 123–48.

Markowitz, S. and Grossman, M. (1998) Alcohol regulation and domestic violence towards children. *Contemporary Economic Policy,* 16, 309–20.

Markowitz, S. and Grossman, M. (2000) The effects of beer taxes on physical child abuse. *Journal of Health Economics,* 19, 271–82.

Marmot, M. (2004) Evidence based policy of policy based evidence? (Editorial) *British Medical Journal,* 328, 906–7.

Martin, A. (2005) Police pledge to target underage drinking culprits. *Northern Constitution,* October 26th, 1.

Mass Observation (1943, 1987) *The Pub and the People.* London: Cresset Library.

Mathews, S. and Richardson, A. (2005) *Findings from the 2004 Offending, Crime and Justice Survey: Alcohol-Related Crime and Disorder.* London: Home Office Research Findings No 261.

Mathias, V. (2005) This is the worst club in Bristol. *Evening Post,* October 4th, 3.

McBride, N. (2005) The evidence base for school drug education interventions. In: Stockwell, T., Gruenewald., P.J., Toumbourou, J.W. and Loxley, W. (eds.) *Preventing Harmful Substance Abuse.* Chichester: Wiley, 101–12.

McCambridge, J. (2005) 24-hour drinking rejected: Ulster's pubs won't open all night. *Belfast Telegraph,* November 1st.

McCormack, S. and Carman, R.S. (1989) Eating motivations and bulimic behaviour among college women *Psychological Reports,* 64, 1163–6.

McDonald, M. (ed) (1994) *Gender, Drink and Drugs: Cross Cultural Perspectives on Women.* Oxford/Providence USA: Berg.

McLynn, F. (1999) *1066: The Year of the Three Battles.* London: Pimlico.

Meikle, J. (2005) Surge in consumption as oral cancer cases increase. *Guardian,* November 16th, 4.

Midford, R. and McBride, N. (2004) Alcohol education in schools. In: Heather, N. and Stockwell, T. (eds.) The *Essential Handbook of Treatment and Prevention of Alcohol Problems.* West Sussex: John Wiley, pp.299–319.

Miller, P. (1997) Family structure, personality, drinking, smoking and illicit drug use: A study of UK teenagers. *Drug and Alcohol Dependence,* 45, 121–9.

Miller, P. and Plant, M.A. (1996) Drinking, smoking and illicit drug use amongst 15–16 year olds: A UK study. *British Medical Journal,* 313, 394–7.

Miller, P. and Plant, M.A. (1999a) Truancy, perceived school performance, family structure, lifestyle, alcohol, cigarettes and illicit drugs: A study of UK teenagers. *Alcohol & Alcoholism,* 34, 886–93.

Miller, P. and Plant, M.A. (1999b) Use and perceived ease of obtaining illicit drugs amongst teenagers in urban, suburban and rural schools: A UK study. *Journal of Substance Use,* 4, 24–8.

Miller, P. and Plant, M.A. (2001a) Drinking and smoking among 15 and 16 year olds in the United Kingdom: A re-examination, *Journal of Substance Use,* 5, 285–9.

Miller, P. and Plant, M.A. (2001b) *Drinking, Smoking and Illicit Drug Use amongst 15 and 16 year old School Students in Northern Ireland,* (Report for Department of Health, Social Services and Public Safety, Belfast), Edinburgh: Alcohol & Health Research Centre.

Miller, P., and Plant, M.A. (2002) Heavy cannabis use among UK teenagers: An exploration. *Drug and Alcohol Dependence*, **65**, 235–42.

Miller, P. and Plant, M.A. (2003a) Teenage beverage preferences: Risk and responses. *Health, Risk and Society* **5**, 3–10.

Miller, P. and Plant, M.A. (2003b) The family, peer influences and substance use among UK teenagers. *Journal of Substance Use*, **8**, 19–26.

Miller, P. and Plant, M.A. (2005) Did your parents teach you to drink? Paper presented at *International Conference on Wet Youth Cultures*, Copenhagen, August 29–30th.

Miller, P., Plant, M.A., Choquet, M., and Ledoux, S. (2002) Cigarettes, alcohol, drugs and self-esteem: A comparison of 15–16 year olds from France and the United Kingdom. *Journal of Substance Use*, **7**, 71–7.

Miller, P., Plant, M.L., and Plant, M.A. (2005) Spreading out or concentrating weekly consumption: Alcohol problems and other consequences within a UK population sample, *Alcohol & Alcoholism*, **40**: 461–468.

Mohler-Kuo M., Dowdall, G., Koss, M and Weschler, H. (2004) Correlates of rape while intoxicated in a sample of college women, *Journal of Studies on Alcohol*, **65**, 37–45.

Mohr A.F. (2000) Adolescent substance-abuse: Vulnerability and protective factors from a developmental perspective *Dissertation Abstracts International Section A: Humanities & Social Sciences* **60**, 7-A: 2373

Moloney, M. (1995) Random breath testing in the State of Victoria, Australia. In: Kloeden, C.N. and Mclean, A.J. (eds.) *Alcohol, Drugs and Traffic Safety, Volume 2*. Australia: NHMRC, Road Accident Research Unit, pp.823–7.

Moore, D (1992) *Has the Emperor no clothes? The NHTA report on Lowering the BAC limit in California*, Washington, DC.: The American Beverage Institute.

Moore, M. and Cooke, P.J. (1995) *Habit and Heterogeneity in the Youthful Demand for Alcohol.* Cambridge, Massachusetts, National Bureau of Economic Research, Working Paper 5152.

Moorhouse (1882) *The effect of alcohol on the blood.* Read at the Conference of British Temperance Association, London.

Morgan J.F., Reid F., and Lacey J.H. (1999) The SCOFF questionnaire: Assessment of a new screening tool for eating disorders. *British Medical Journal* **319**, 1467–8.

Morgan, M. (2004) Personal communication.

Mullins, L.J. (2005) *Management and Organisational Behaviour.* Harlow: Prentice Hall.

Musto, D. (1997) Alcohol control in historical perspective, In: Plant, M.A., Single, E. and Stockwell, T. (eds.) *Alcohol: Minimising the Harm: What Works?* London: Free Association Books, pp.10–28.

Naimi, T.S., Lipscomb L.E., Brewer R.D. and Gilbert B, C. (2003) Binge drinking in the preconception period and the risk of unintended pregnancy: Implications for women and their children. *Pediatrics*, **111**, 1136–41.

National Assembly for Wales (2000) *Tackling Substance Misuse in Wales: a Partnership Approach.* Cardiff, National Assembly for Wales.

National Centre for Social Research/National Foundation for Educational Research (2005) *Smoking, Drinking & Drug Use among Young People in England in 2004*, online summary, March 9th, National Centre for Social Research/National Foundation for Educational Research.

National Centre for Social Research/National Foundation for Educational Research (2005) *Smoking, Drinking and Drug Use among Young People in England in 2004.* London: National Centre for Social Research/National Foundation for Educational Research.

The National Organisation for Fetal Alcohol Syndrome-UK (NOFAS-UK) (2005) Should the Government put warning labels on alcohol? (YOUGOV Poll). London: NOFAS-UK.

Newburn, T. and Shiner, M. (2001) *Teenage Kicks? Young People and Alcohol: A Review of the Literature.* York: Joseph Rowntree Foundation.

Newell, C. and Watt, H. (2005) Tories turn to prayer in final effort to halt 24-hour drinking, *Sunday Times,* October 9th, 1.2.

Newman, C. (2005) Backtrack on drink laws. *Financial Times,* September 17th, 1.

Nicholson Committee (2003) *Review of Liquor Licensing in Scotland.* Edinburgh: Scottish Executive.

O'Connor, J. (1978) *The Young Drinkers.* London: Tavistock.

O'Malley, P.M. and Wagenaar, A.C. (1981) Effects of minimum drinking age laws on alcohol user, related behaviours and traffic crash involvement among American youth: 1976–1987. *Journal of Studies on Alcohol,* 52, 478–91.

Oaten, M. (2005) Personal communication.

Obote, I. (2005) The international picture. Paper presented at international conference on *Alcohol Problems: Prevention & Treatment,* Bristol, November 11th.

Observer (2002) News in Brief: Pubs reject 24-hour boozing, *Observer,* January 30th, 5.

Oesterle, S., Hill, K.G., Hawkins, J.D., Guo, J., Catalano, R.F. and Abbott, R.D. (2004) Adolescent heavy episodic drinking trajectories and health in young adulthood. *Journal of Studies on Alcohol,* 65, 204–12.

Office of National Statistics (2005) *General Household Survey 2003* (online). London: Office of National Statistics.

Olafsdottír, H. (2003) Perceptions of Drinking and Public Disorder. Presentation given at the 29th Annual Alcohol Symposium of the Kettil Bruun Society for Social and Epidemiological Research on Alcohol, Krakow, Poland June 2–6.

Olafsdottír, H. (2005) Personal communication.

Oliver, J. (2005a) This is the expert who is behind Labour's 24-hour drinking law, *Mail on Sunday,* August 21st, 4–5.

Oliver, J. (2005b) Now it's 24-hour drinking for kids. *Mail on Sunday,* August 28th, 1.

Oliver, J. (2005) Revealed: How 24-hour drinking laws were drawn up over lunch at alcohol industry's HQ, *Mail on Sunday,* September 4th, 13.

Office of National Statistics (2005) *Results from the 2003 General Household Survey,* ONS online.

Österberg, E. (1995) Do alcohol prices affect consumption and related problems? In Edwards, G. (ed.) *Alcohol and Public Policy: Evidence and Issues.* Oxford: Oxford University Press, 145–63.

Österberg, E. and Karlson,T. (Eds.) (2002) *Alcohol Policies in EU Member States and Norway.* Helsinki: National Research and Development Centre for Welfare and Health.

Parker, H., Aldridge, J. and Measham, F. (1998) *Illegal Leisure: The Normalisation of Adolescent Drug Use.* London: Routledge.

Parker, H. and Egginton, R. (2002) Adolescent recreational alcohol and drug careers gone wrong: Developing a strategy for reducing risks and harms. *International Journal of Drug Policy,* 13, 4119–423.

Parker, H. and Williams, L. (2001) Intoxicated weekends: Young adults' work hard, play hard lifestyles, public health and public disorder. *Drugs: Education, Prevention and Policy*, 40, 345–68.

Parks, K.A., Miller, B.A., Collins, R.L. and Zetes-Zanatta, L. (1998) Women's descriptions of drinking in bars: Reasons and risks. *Sex Roles*, 38, 701–17.

Parliamentary Office of Science and Technology, (2005) *Binge Drinking and Public Health*. London: Parliamentary Office of Science and Technology, July, Bulletin Number 244.

Partridge B. (2002) *A History of Orgies*. London: Prion Books Ltd.

Pearlman, N. (2005) What's your daughter drinking tonight? *Daily Mail*, September 23rd, 26–7.

Phipps R. (2005) Addiction within a Northern Ireland context. Paper presented at International Addictions Conference Exploring Research, Policy and Practice, Jordanstown Campus, University of Ulster, September 7th.

Pitkänen, T., Lyyra, A-L and Pulkkenen, L. (2004) Age of onset of drinking and the use of alcohol in adulthood: A follow-up study from age 8–42 for females and males. *Addiction*, 100, 652–61.

Pitman, D.J. and Raskin-White, H. (eds.) (1991) *Society, Culture and Drinking Patterns Re-Examined*. New Brunswick, New Jersey: Rutgers Center of Alcohol Studies.

Plant, E.J. and Plant, M.A. (2005) A leap in the dark? Lessons for the United Kingdom from past extensions of bar opening hours. (commentary) *International Journal of Drug Policy*, 16: 363–368.

Plant, M.A. (1999) ESPAD: The European School Survey Project on Alcohol & Other Drugs. *Alcohol Update*. Glasgow: Scottish Council on Alcohol, 40, 2–3.

Plant, M.A. (2000) Young people and alcohol use. In: Aggleton, P., Hurry, J., and Warwick, I. (eds.) *Young People and Mental Health*. London: Wiley, pp. 13–28.

Plant, M.A. (2001) Learning by experiment. In: Grant, M. (ed.) *Learning about Drinking*. International Center for Alcohol Policies Series on Alcohol in Society, Philadelphia: Brunner/Mazel 129–146.

Plant, M.A. (2004a) The Alcohol Harm Reduction Strategy for England: Overdue final report omits much that was useful in interim report. *British Medical Journal* 328, 905–6.

Plant, M.A. (2004b) Reducing the pressure to drink: An interview with Dr Christopher Clayson. *Alcohol & Alcoholism*, 39, 5–7.

Plant, M.A. and Cameron, D. (eds.) (2000) *The Alcohol Report*. London: Free Association Books.

Plant, M.A. and Miller, P. (2001a) Teenage drinking in Europe: ESPAD 1999, *Straight Talk* (Alcohol Concern Magazine). London: Alcohol Concern, 16, 3–4.

Plant, M.A. and Miller, P. (2001b) UK youth are heaviest drug users in Europe-again. *Substance Misuse Bulletin* 14, 2–3.

Plant, M.A. and Miller, P. (2001c) Young people and alcohol: An international insight. *Alcohol & Alcoholism*, 36, 513–15.

Plant, M.A. and Miller, P. (2001d) The 1999 European School Survey Project on Alcohol & other Drugs. London: Alcohol Education & Research Council.

Plant, M.A. and Plant, M.L. (1992) *Risktakers: Alcohol, Drugs, Sex and Youth*, London: Tavistock.

Plant, M.A., and Plant, M.L. (2001) Young people and alcohol, *Nursing Times Research* 6: 887–896.

Plant, M.A. and Plant, M.L. (2004) Binge drinking: What's happening? Presentation at Binge Drinking: Problems and Responses, an international conference, Bristol, November 26th.

Plant, M.A. Kreitman, N., Miller, T., and Duffy, J. (1977) Observing public drinking. *Journal of Studies on Alcohol*, 38, 867–80.

Plant, M.A., Peck, D., and Samuel, E. (1985) *Alcohol, Drugs and School-Leavers*. London: Tavistock.

Plant, M.A., Plant, M.L., and Nichol, P. (1994) No such thing as a safe glass. *British Medical Journal*, 308, 1237–8.

Plant, M.A., Single, E., and Stockwell, T. (eds.) (1997) *Alcohol: Minimising the Harm: What Works?* London: Free Association Books.

Plant, M.A., Plant, M.L., Thornton, C. and Garretsen, H. (2000) Consequences: Patterns and trends. In: Plant, M.A. and Cameron, D. (eds.) *The Alcohol Report*. London: Free Association Books, pp.130–9.

Plant, M.A., Miller, P. and Plant, M.L. (2005) Trends in drinking, smoking and illicit drug use among 15 and 16 year olds in the United Kingdom (1995–2003). *Journal of Substance Use*, 10: 331–339.

Plant, M.L. (1985) *Women, Drinking and Pregnancy*. London: Tavistock.

Plant, M.L. (1997) *Women and Alcohol: Contemporary and Historical Perspectives*. London: Free Association Books.

Plant, M.L. and Plant, M.A. (2001) Heavy drinking by young British women gives cause for concern. *British Medical Journal*, 323, 1183.

Plant, M.L., Abel, E., and Guerri, C. (1999) Alcohol and Pregnancy, In: Macdonald, I. (ed.) Health *Issues Related to Alcohol Consumption*. London: Blackwell Science, pp.181–214.

Plant, M.L., Plant, M.A., and Mason, W. (2002a) Drinking, smoking and illicit drug use amongst British adults: Gender differences explored. *Journal of Substance Use* 7, 24–33.

Plant, M.L., Plant, M.A., and Mason, W. (2002b) People who enjoy drinking: Findings from a Survey of British adults. *The Drug and Alcohol Professional*, 2, 26–37.

Plant, M.L., Miller, P., and Plant, M.A. (2004) Childhood and adult sexual abuse: relationships with alcohol and other drug use. *Child Abuse Review*, 13, 200–14

Plant, M.L. Miller, P., and Plant, M.A. (2005) The relationship between alcohol consumption and problem behaviours: Gender differences among British adults. *Journal of Substance Use*, 10, 22–30.

Plant, M.L., Miller, P., and Plant, M.A. (submitted) Alcohol consumption, sexual abuse and relationships with a partner. *Journal of substance use.*

Plant, M.L., Plant, M.A., and Miller, P. (2005) Childhood and adult sexual abuse: Relationships with addictive or problem behaviours and health. *Journal of Addictive Diseases*, 24, 25–38.

Porter, R. (1985) The drinking man's disease: The prehistory of drinking in Georgian Britain. *British Journal of Addiction*, 80: 385–396.

Poulin, C. and Nicholson, J. (2005) Should harm minimization as an approval to adolescent substance use be embraced by junior and senior high schools? *International Journal of Drug Policy*, 16: 403–414.

Powell, J., Plant, M.A., Steriu, A., and Miller, P. (2004) *Drinking, Smoking and Illicit Drug Use Amongst 15 & 16 Year Old School Students in the Isle of Man: A Report for the Department of Health & Social Security, Douglas, Isle of Man*. Bristol: University of the West of England.

Powell, J., Steriu, A., Plant, M.A., and Miller (2006) Drinking, smoking and illicit drug use among 15 and 16 year olds in the Isle of Man. *Journal of Substance Use*, 11: 1–9.

Press Association (2005) Jowell opposed to 24-hour drinking, January 16th.

Purcell N (1994) *Women and Wine in Ancient Rome* In McDonald, M. (ed) *Gender, Drink and Drugs: Cross Cultural Perspectives on Women.* Oxford/Providence USA Berg.

Ragnarsdottír, P, Kjartansdottír, Ä., and Davídsdottír, S. (2002) Effect of Extended Alcohol Serving-Hours in Reykjavík. In Room, R. (ed.) *The Effects of Nordic Alcohol Policies: what happens to drinking and harm when alcohol controls change?* Helsinki, Finland: NAD Publication 42, pp.145–54.

Ratcliffe, W.D. and Nutter, R.W. (1979) *Drinking in Edmonton Taverns and Lounges.* Final report to the Alberta Liquor Licensing Board.

Rehm, J. (1999) Draining the ocean to prevent shark attacks? *Nordic Studies on Alcohol and Drugs,* 16, 46–54.

Renault, S. and de Logeril, M. (1992) Wine, cigarettes, platelets and the French paradox for coronary heart disease, Lancet, 339: 1523–1536.

Rehm, J., Room, R., van den Brink, W. and Jacobi, F. (2005) Alcohol use disorders in European Union countries and Norway, *Neuropsychopharmacology* 15, 377–88.

Richardson, A. and Budd, T. (2003) *Alcohol, Crime and Disorder: A Study of Young Adults.* Home Office Research Study Number 263. London: Home Office.

Rickert V.I., Vaughan R.D. and Wiemann C.M. (2002) Adolescent dating violence and date rape. *Current Opinions in Obstetrics and Gynecology,* 14, 495–500.

Rimm, E.B., Klatsky, A., Grobbee, D. and Stampher, M.J. (1996) Review of moderate alcohol consumption and reduced risk of coronary heart disease, *British Medical Journal,* 312: 731–736.

Robbins, T. (2005) Do You Want This 24 Hours a Day? *Sunday Times,* January 16th 21.

Room, R., (1980) Concepts and strategies in the prevention of alcohol-related problems. *Contemporary Drug Problems,* 9, 85–106.

Room, R. (1984) Alcohol control policy and public health. *American Review of Public Health,* 5, 293–317.

Room, R. (2002) *The Effects of Nordic Alcohol Policies.* Nordic Council for Alcohol and Drug Research, NAD Publication 42. Helsinki: Nordic Council for Alcohol and Drug Research.

Room, R. (2004a) Disabling the public interest: Alcohol strategies and policies for England. *Addiction,* 99, 1083–9.

Room, R. (2004b) The alcohol industry & British research funding, Kettil Bruun Society list serve. June 18th (kbs-list@listserve.nodak.edu).

Room, R., Romelsjö, A., and Mäkelä, P. (2002) Impacts of Alcohol Policy: The Nordic experience. In Room, R. (ed.) *The Effects of Nordic Alcohol Policies: what happens to drinking and harm when alcohol controls change?* Helsinki, Finland: NAD Publication 42, pp.167–74.

Rosenberg, L., Slone, D. and Shapiro, G. (1981) Alcoholic beverage and myocardical infraction in young women. *American Journal of Public Health* 71: 82–85.

Rowntree, J. and Sherwell, A. (1999) *The Temperance Problem and Social Reform.* London: Hodder and Stoughton.

Royal College of General Practitioners (1986) *Alcohol: A Balanced View.* London: Tavistock.

Royal College of Physicians (1987) *Alcohol: A Great and Growing Evil: The Medical Consequences of Alcohol Abuse.* London: Tavistock.

Royal College of Psychiatrists (1979) *Alcohol and Alcoholism.* London: Tavistock.

Royal College of Psychiatrists (1986) *Alcohol: Our Favourite Drug.* London: Tavistock.

Rydon, P. and Stockwell, T. (1997) Local regulation for licensed premises. In: Plant, M.A., Single, E. and Stockwell, T. (eds.) *Alcohol: Minimising the Harm: What Works?* London: Free Association Books, pp.211–29.

St Leger, A.G., Cochrane A.L. and Moore E. (1979) Factors associated with cardiac mortality in developed countries, *Lancet* 1: 1017–1020.

Saffer, H. and Grossman, M. (1987) Beer taxes, the legal drinking age, and youth motor vehicle fatalities. *Journal of Legal Studies*, 16, 351–74.

Saltz, R.E. (1997) Prevention where alcohol is sold and consumed: server intervention and responsible beverage service, In: Plant, M.A., Single, E. and Stockwell, T. (eds.) *Alcohol: Minimising the Harm: What Works?* London: Free Association Books, pp.72–84.

Savill, R. (2005) Pub appeal costs taxpayer £30,000. *Daily Telegraph*, November 23rd, 12.

Schaps, E., Dibartolo, R., Moskowitz, J., Bailey, C.G., and Churgin, G. (1981) A review of 127 drug abuse prevention program evaluations. *Journal of Drug Issues*, 11, 17–43.

Scotsman (2005a) Time for some sober reflection, (Editorial), *Scotsman*, November 17th, 31.

Scotsman (2005b) Fresh calls to delay 24-hour drinking plans, *Scotsman* April 1st.

Scottish Executive (2002) *Plan for Action on Alcohol Problems.* Edinburgh: Scottish Parliament.

Scottish Executive (2002a) *Consultation with Children and Young People on the Scottish Executive's Plan for Action on Alcohol Misuse.* Edinburgh: Scottish Executive.

Scottish Executive (2002b) *Omnibus Survey: Testing Public Opinion on Licensing Law and Alcohol Consumptio*n. http:www.scotland.gov.uk/library5/justice/ostp-01.asp

Scottish Executive (2003) The Nicholson Committee: Review of Liquor Licensing Law in Scotland. http://www.scotland.gov.uk/library5/society/flllm-00.asp

Scottish Executive (2004) The Licensing (Scotland) Bill: A Consultation on Liquor Licensing. http://www.scotland.gov.uk/consultations/justice/lbcll

Scottish Executive (2005) Licensing Scotland Bill Published. http://www.scotland.gov.uk/News/releases/2005/03/011059225

Scribner, R.A., MacKinnon, D.P, and Dwyer, J.H. (1995) Risk of assaultive violence and alcohol availability in Los Angeles County. *American Journal of Public Health*, 85, 335–40.

Shadwell, A. (1903) *Drink, Temperance and Legislation.* London: Longmans, Green and Co.

Shadwell, A. (1923) *Drink in 1914–1992, a Lesson in Control.* London: Longmans, Green and Co.

Shakespeare, W. (ca 1605) *Macbeth.*

Shampoo (1996) Girl power, (lyrics by Stanley and Wiggs). *Girl Power,* Food (EMI) Records.

Shepherd, J. (1994) Violent crime: the role of alcohol and new approaches to the prevention of injury. *Alcohol and Alcoholism*, 29, 5–10.

Shepherd, J., Irish, M., Scully, C. and Leslie, I. (1988) Alcohol intoxication and severity of injury in victims of assault. *British Medical Journal*, 296, 1299.

Shepherd, K.J. And Brinkley, J. (1996) The relationship between alcohol consumption and alcohol intoxication, stressors an injury in urban violence, *British Journal of Criminology*, 36, 546–66.

Shiman L.L. (1988) *Crusade against Drink in Victorian England* London: MacMillan Press.

Shipman, T. (2005) Drink law retreat, *Daily Mail*, September 17th, 4.

Single, E. (1982) Intercorporate connections of the alcohol industry in Canada. *Contemporary Drug Problems*, 11, 545–67.

Single, E., Robson, L., Xie, X., and Rehm, J. (1998) The economic costs of alcohol, tobacco and illicit drugs in Canada, 1992. *Addiction*, **93**, 991–1006.

Skog, O-J. (1986) Long waves of alcohol consumption: A social network perspective on cultural change. *Social Networks*, **8**, 1–32.

Skog, O-J. (1999) The prevention paradox revisited. *Addiction*, **94**, 751–7.

Skog, O-J. (2001a) Alcohol consumption and overall accident mortality in 14 European countries, *Addiction*, **96**, (S1), S35–S47.

Skog, O-J. (2001b) Alcohol consumption and mortality rates from traffic accidents, accidental falls, and other accidents in 14 European countries. *Addiction*, **96** (S1), S49–S58.

Slack, J. (2005a) Jowell slapped down by police. *Daily Mail*, November 16th, 6–7.

Slack, J. (2005b) Ladettes drink before they go out. *Daily Express* January 22nd, 5.

Slack, J. (2005c) Police anger over delays in 24-hour drinking powers. *Daily Mail*, November 21st, 6.

Slack, J. (2005d) 700 pubs, clubs and shops get a 24-hour licence. *Daily Mail*, November 15th, 8.

Slack, J. (2005e) Drunken madness, *Daily Express*, November 22nd, p.5.

Slack, J. and Hickley, M. (2005a) Taxpayers to pick up a £70m tab for 24-hour licensing. *Daily Mail*, November 22nd, 15.

Slack, J. and Hickley, M. (2005b) Drinks crime: it will go up. *Daily Mail*, November 16th, 1.

Sloan, F.A., Reilly, B.A., and Schenzer, C. (1994) Effects of prices, civil and criminal sanctions, and law enforcement on alcohol-related mortality. *Journal of Studies on Alcohol*, **55**, 454–65.

Smart, T. (1974) The effect of licensing restrictions during 1914–19 on drunkenness and liver cirrhosis deaths in Britain. *British Journal of Addiction*, **69**, 109–21.

Smith, D. (1988) Effect on traffic accidents of introducing flexible hotel trading hours in Tasmania, Australia. *British Journal of Addiction*, **83**, 219–22.

Sommer, R. (1965) The isolated drinker in the Edmonton beer parlor. *Quarterly Journal of Studies on Alcohol*, **26**, 95–110.

Sommer, R. (1969) *Personal Space: The Behavioral Basis of Design*. Englewood Cliffs: Prentice Hall.

Sparrow, A. (2005) New pub law 'will mean fewer police for day duty. *Daily Telegraph*, August 11th, 1.

Spender Q. (2004) Assessment of adolescent self harm. *Current Paediatrics* 15, 120–6.

Stampfer, M.J., Colditz, G.A., Willett, W.C. *et al.* (1988) A prospective a study of moderate alcohol consumption and the risk of coronary disease and stroke in women. *New England Journal of Medicine*, **319**, 267–73.

Stenius, K. (2004) Conflicting interest. *Nordic Studies on Alcohol and Drugs*, 21, 108–10.

Sternberg, E. (1994) *Just Business*. London: Little, Brown.

Stewart, K. and Sweedler, B.M. (1997) Driving under the influence. In: Plant, M.A., Single, E., and Stockwell, T. (**eds.**) *Alcohol: Minimising the Harm: What Works?* London: Free Association Books, pp.126–42.

Stockwell, T., Gruenewald., P.J., Toumbourou, J.W., and Loxley, W. (eds.). (2005) *Preventing Harmful Substance Abuse*. Chichester: Wiley.

Stockwell, T. (2004a) Australian alcohol policy and the public interest: A brief report card. *Drug Policy Review* 23, 377–9.

Stockwell, T. (2004b) Harm minimisation. Presentation at Binge Drinking: Problems and Responses, an International Conference. Bristol, November 26th.

Stockwell, T. and Single, E. (1997) Standard unit labelling of alcohol containers. In: Plant, M.A., Single, E. and Stockwell, T. (eds.) *Alcohol: Minimising the Harm: What Works?* London: Free Association Books, pp.85–104.

Storch, R. (1977) The problem of working-class leisure: Some roots of middle class moral reform in the industrial North, 1825–50. In: Donajgrodzsdki, A.P. (ed.) *Social Control in Nineteenth Century Britain.* London: Croom Helm, pp.138–62.

Stratford, N. and Roth, W. (1999) *The 1988 Youth Lifestyles Survey.* London: National Centre for Social Research.

Sullivan, W.C. (1899) A note on the influence of maternal inebriety on the offspring. *Journal of Mental Science* 45, 489–503.

Sussex Police (1987) *Sussex Police Liquor Licensing Project, Brighton: 1986–1987, a project to Identify and Reduce Alcohol-related Crime.* Brighton: Sussex Police.

Sutton, M. and Godfrey, C. (1995) A grouped data regression approach to estimating economic and social influences on individual drinking behaviour. *Health Economics,* 4, 237–47.

Temperance Tract (1870s) *Nuts to Crack for Moderate Drinkers.* (unsigned)

Temperance Song (1880s) The cold water templar.

Tether, P. and Robinson, D. (1986) *Preventing Alcohol Problems,* London: Tavistock.

The Telegraph Online (2005) Doctors Say 24-Hour Pub Opening Will Cost NHS Millions. January 5th. http://news.telegraph.co.uk/core/Content/displayPrintable.jhtml; sessionid-IX4EXU23

Thom, B. (1999) *Dealing with Drink.* London: Free Association Books.

Thom, B. Herring, R., and Judd, A. (1999) Identifying alcohol-related harm and young drinkers: The role of accident and emergency departments. *Alcohol and Alcoholism,* 34, 1475–87.

Thompson, A. (2005) Next week 24-hour drinking becomes legal. But what safeguards are in place to protect vulnerable youngsters? *Daily Mail,* November 16th, 26–7.

Thornton, S. (1996) *Club Cultures: Music, Media and Subcultural Capital.* Middletown, Connecticut: Wesleyan University Press.

Tighe, A. (2005) Personal communication.

Times (2005) Populus Poll. *Times,* September 5–8th. http://64.233.161.104/ search?q= cache:4osRuQPfpmkJ: www.populuslimited.com/poll

Tobler, N. (1986) Meta-analysis of 143 adolescent drug abuse prevention programs: Quantitative results of program participants compared to a control or comparison group. *Journal of Drug Issues,* 16, 537–67.

Toussaint Samat M. (1994) *History of Food* Bell, A., (trans). Oxford: Blackwell Publishers.

Townshend, J. and Duka, T. (2005) Binge drinking, cognitive performance and mood in a population of young social drinkers. *Alcoholism: Clinical & Experimental Research* 29, 317–25.

Toynbee, P. (2005) Only raising prices will end our love affair with booze. *Guardian,* August 24th, 20.

Transportation Research Board (1994) *The Nature of and Reasons for the Worldwide Decline in Drinking and Driving,* Transport Research Circular, Number 422, April. Washington, DC: Transportation Research Board.

Travis, A. (2005a) Drink law rethink urged after rise in violence. *Guardian*, October 21st, 4.

Travis, A. (2005b) New powers to tackle drunken troublemakers. *Guardian*, September 30th, 1.

Travis, A. (2005c) Whitehall clash in the battle to beat bingers. *Guardian*, January 22nd 10.

Travis, A. (2005d) Public opposes licensing changes. *Guardian*, January 26th, 10.

Travis, A. (2005e) Levy on pubs to police yobs. *Guardian*, January 21st, 4.

Travis, A., Muir, H. and Cowan, R. (2005) Government admits new drinking hours could lead to increase in offences. *Guardian*, November 23rd, 3.

Treno, A.J., Lee, J.P., Freisler, B., Remer, L.G. and Guenwald, P.J. (2005) Application of evidence-based approaches to community interventions, In: Stockwell, T., Gruenewald., P.J., Toumbourou, J.W. and Loxley, W. (eds.) *Preventing Harmful Substance Abuse.* Chichester: Wiley, p.177–90.

Trotter, T. (1804) *An Essay Medical, Philosophical and Chemical on Drunkenness*, Boston, Mass: Bradford and Read. (Reprinted 1981 by New York: Arno Press).

Turnbull, D. and Oliver, J. (2005) 24-hour pub MPs' £200, 000 free bar, *Mail on Sunday*, August 14th, 8–9.

Turner, E.S. (1950) *Roads to Ruin. The Shocking History of Social Reform.* London: Michael Joseph Ltd.

Turner, I. (2004) Expert Calls Time on Booze Strategy. *Bristol Evening Post*, November 26th, 22.

Twain, S. (1998) Man, I feel like a woman. (Lyrics by Twain, S. and Lang, R.). *Come on Over*, Mercury Records.

UKATT Research Team (2005a) Cost effectiveness of treatment for alcohol problems: Findings of the UK alcohol treatment trial. *British Medical Journal* 331, 544–8.

UKATT Research Team (2005b) Effectiveness of treatment for alcohol problems: Findings of the UK alcohol treatment trial, *British Medical Journal* 331, 541–4.

Ungoed-Thomas, J. and Winnett, R. (2005) Councils rebel on late-night drinking laws, *Sunday Times* August 14th, 10.

Ungoed-Thomas, J. and Swinford, S. (2005) Late licenses to fuel £500m alcohol boom, *Sunday Times*, November 20th, 1.

United Kingdom Parliament (2005) Hansard Debates for 25th January column 167–169. http://www.publications.uk/pa/cm200405/cmhansrd/cm050125/debtext

Van Oers, V. and Garretsen, H. (1993) Geographic relationship between alcohol use, bars, liquor shops and traffic injuries in Rotterdam. *Journal of Studies on Alcohol*, 54, 739–44.

Velleman, R., Copello, A. and Maslin, J. (eds.) (1998) *Living with Drink*. London: Longman.

Velleman, R. and Orford, J. (1999) *Risk and Resilience: Adults who were the children of problem drinkers*. Amsterdam: Harwood Academic Publishers.

Vingilis, E., McLeod, A., Seeley, J., Mann, R., Bierness, D., Compton, C. (2005) Road safety impact of extended drinking hours in Ontario. *Accident, Analysis & Prevention* 37, 549–56.

Voas, R.B., Tippetts, A.S., and Fell, J. (1999) *United States Limits Drinking by Youth under 21: Does it Reduce Fatal Crash Involvements?* Paper presented at the annual meeting of the Association for the Advancement of Automotive Medicine, Barcelona, Spain.

Wagenaar, A.C. and Maybee, R.G. (1986) Legal minimum drinking age in Texas: Effects of an increase from 18 to 19. *Journal of Safety Research*, 17, 165–78.

Walker, A., Maher, J., Coullthard, M., Goddard, E. and Thomas, M. (2001) *Living in Britain: Results from the 2000 General Household Survey.* London: The Stationery Office.

Waller, M. (2000) *1700: Scenes from London Life,* New York: Four Walls Eight Windows.

Wallin, E. and Andréasson, S. (2005) Effects of a community action programme on problems related to alcohol consumption in licensed premises. In: Stockwell, T., Gruenewald., P.J., Toumbourou, J.W., and Loxley, W. (eds.) *Preventing Harmful Substance Abuse.* Chichester: Wiley, pp. 207–24.

Walters, S. and Lewis, J. (2005) Exposed: Mandarin ally of alcohol bosses. *Mail on Sunday,* 1,8–9.

Waring, M.L. and Sperr, I. (1982) A comparative study of male and female bartenders: Their potential for assisting in the prevention of alcohol abuse. *Journal of Alcohol and Drug Education,* **28,** 1–11.

Warner J. (1994) Resolv'd to drink no more: addiction as a preindustrial construct. *Journal of Studies on Alcohol* 55, 685–91.

Warner, J. (2003) *Craze: Gin and Debauchery in an Age of Reason.* London: Profile.

Warner R.H. and Rosett H.L. (1975) The effects of drinking on offspring; an historical survey of the American British literature. *Journal of Studies on Alcohol* **36,** 1395–1420

Webb, S. and Webb, B. (1963) *History of the Liquor Licensing Laws in England.* London: Frank Cass.

Wells, S. (2004) Reducing trouble in bars. Presentation at *Binge Drinking: Problems and Responses,* an international conference, Bristol, November 26th.

Welsh Office (1996) Forward Together: A Strategy to Combat Drug and Alcohol Misuse in Wales. Cardiff: The Welsh Office.

Weschler, H., Seibring, M., Chao-Liu, I. and Ahl, M. (2004) Colleges respond to student binge drinking: Reducing student demand or limiting access, *Journal of American College Health* **52,** 159–68.

White, M. (2005) Police oppose 24-hour drinking, *Guardian,* August 10th, 5

White, M. and Dodd, V. (2005) Ministers cool over drinks ban on public transport. *Guardian,* October 31st, 4.

White, M. and Hencke, D. (2005) Last minute Tory attempt to block 24-hour drinking, *Guardian,* November 16th, 4.

Whitehead, T. (2005a) Binge drink laws in chaos, *Daily Express,* June 20th, 1, 6.

Whitehead, T. (2005b) Blunder mars start of 24-hour drinking, *Daily Express,* November 21st, 15.

Wiederman M.W. and Pryor T. (1996) Substance use and impulsive behaviours among adolescents with eating disorders. *Addictive Behaviours* 21, 269–72.

Wilkinson, H. (1994) *No Turning Back: Generations and the Genderquake.* London: Demos.

Wilkinson, H. (1995) *Generation X and the New Work Ethic.* London: Demos.

Williams, G.P. and Brake, G.T. (1980) *Drink in Great Britain.* London: Edsall.

Williamson, J., Sham, P. and Ball, D. (2003) Binge drinking trends in a UK community-based sample. *Journal of Substance Use* 8, 234–7.

Wilsnack, R.W. and Wilsnack, S.C. (eds.) (1997) *Gender and Alcohol: Individual and Social Perspectives.* New Brunswick, New Jersey: Rutgers Center of Alcohol Studies.

Wilson, P. (1980) *Drinking in England and Wales.* London: HMSO.

Wilson, G.B. (1940) *Alcohol and the Nation: A Contribution to the Study of the Liquor Problem in the United Kingdom.* London: Nicholson and Watson.

Winnet, R. and Leppard, D. (2005) Blunkett's anger over drink laws. *Sunday Times*, January 16th, 1–2.

Winskill P.T. (undated) *The Comprehensive History of the Rise and Progress of the Temperance Reformation. From the Earliest Period to September 1881* Warrington. Winskill

Wintour, P. (2005a) Minister cites support of police chiefs to head off rebellion. *Guardian*, October 11th, 15.

Wintour, P. (2005b) Ministers plan total smoking ban in pubs. *Guardian*, October 10th, 7.

Wintour, P. (2005c) Smoking ban in chaos after cabinet revolt. *Guardian*, October 25th, 4.

Woolfenden, S., Dossetor, D., and Williams, K. (2002) Children and adolescents with acute alcohol intoxication/self-poisoning presenting to the emergency department. *Archives of Pediatrics and Adolescent Medicine* 156, 345–8.

World Health Organization (1994) *European Alcohol Action Plan.* Copenhagen: World Health Organization.

World Health Organization (1996) *Alcohol-Less is Better.* Copenhagen: World Health Organization, Regional Publications, European Series number 70.

Worthington, S. (2005) Stores warned over under-age drinkers. *Mail on Sunday*, October 23rd, 50.

York, J.L., Welte, J., Hirsch, J., Hoffman, J.H. and Barnes, G. (2004) Association of age of first drink with current alcohol drinking variables in a national general population sample. *Alcohol, Clinical and Experimental Research*, 28, 1379–87.

Ystgaard, M., Hestetun, I., Loet, M. and Mehlum, L. (2004) Is there a specific relationship between childhood sexual and physical abuse and repeated suicidal behaviour? *Child Abuse and Neglect*, 28: 863–875.

Zarun, S. (1978) The well-scrubbed face on the barroom floor. *MacLean's Magazine*, March, 62–3.

Index